COMPANION TO
NEONATAL MEDICINE

'At first the infant, mewling and puking in the nurse's arms'

As You Like It, Act II, Sc. vii

COMPANION TO
NEONATAL MEDICINE

Victor G. Daniels
Christ's College
Cambridge

Christopher L-H. Huang
New Hall
Cambridge

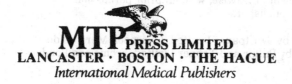

MTP **PRESS LIMITED**
LANCASTER · BOSTON · THE HAGUE
International Medical Publishers

Published in the UK and Europe by
MTP Press Limited
Falcon House
Lancaster, England

British Library Cataloguing in Publication Data

Daniels, Victor G.
  Companion to neonatal medicine.
  1. Infants (Newborn)
  I. Title   II. Huang, Christopher L.-H.
  618.92'01   RJ251

  ISBN 0-85200-380-3

Published in the USA by
MTP Press
A division of Kluwer Boston Inc
190 Old Derby Street
Hingham, MA 02043, USA

Typeset by Swiftpages Limited, Liverpool, Merseyside
Printed by Butler and Tanner Limited, Frome and London

Contents

Preface

This book is one of a series of three volumes summarizing the principles of obstetrics, gynaecology and neonatal medicine. It provides a clear and systematic summary of the principles of neonatal medicine in synoptic form. Where appropriate, fundamentals of related biochemistry, physiology and pathology are also considered. It is primarily directed at undergraduate medical students and senior nurses, but material useful as reference to doctors revising for further qualifications has been included. It should be particularly useful for staff working on special care baby units. Although much of the content is organized in the form of lists, this book differs from the usual 'list' book in that coverage is full and systematic. Therefore, it serves both as a text and a revision aid. Thus the text has been organized into the following subheadings, where appropriate: definitions, aetiology, pathophysiology, clinical features, differential diagnosis, investigations, treatment and prognosis. The format employed should also assist those preparing for examinations. Useful diagnostic lists are also provided. Illustrations have been specially prepared in the form of explanatory line drawings that are simple, and easy to memorize and reproduce. Although drug dosages were checked with care, changes in medical practice make it advisable to verify regimes and doses with

7

8   *Companion to neonatal medicine*

the latest prescribing information and the British or US pharmacopoeia before use.

We are very grateful to Dr Ann Greenough for detailed reading and criticism of the text through all its stages. Fiona Hake prepared the illustrations. Our thanks also to Mrs Kay Serby and Mrs Pat Smith who transformed our illegible handwriting into manuscript. Finally, we acknowledge the kind help of Merrell Pharmaceuticals, and in particular Mr P. D. V. Cannon, for assistance towards production of artwork. All errors, however, remain the responsibility of the authors. We would welcome comments and suggestions for future editions.

Cambridge   VICTOR G. DANIELS
Easter 1982   CHRISTOPHER L.-H. HUANG

1

Development of the Fetus

Embryology concerns the events beginning with fertilization of the female germ cell (the ovum) by the male germ cell (spermatozoon), and ending with the birth of the child. This is the result of two fundamental processes:

1 Growth: Involves increase in size due to cell division or enlargement. It is dependent upon availability of adequate nutrition

2 Differentiation: This is where groups of cells acquire, in the course of development, particular characteristics which enable them to carry out a specialized function

All human somatic cells possess 46 chromosomes. Of these one pair are sex chromosomes, denoted as XX in female and XY in male. During meiosis, all ova receive one X chromosome but spermatozoa may receive either an X or a Y chromosome. At fertilization, if the fusing spermatozoon contains an X chromosome, a female child results, and if it contains a Y, a male child results.

After fusion, as the zygote passes down the Fallopian tube it rapidly subdivides, producing:

1 A morula – a solid ball of cells, and then

2   The blastula – a hollow ball of cells. The blastula differentiates into an outer cell layer, which will form the trophoblast, and the inner cell layer, which will form the embryo

IMPLANTATION

Between 7 and 9 days after ovulation the blastula (which now consists of about 200 cells) becomes embedded into endometrium, usually in the fundus or cornua. Implantation is conditional upon the endometrium having been suitably prepared, in the secretory phase of the menstrual cycle. The endometrium surrounds the blastula and can be divided into

1   Decidua basalis, which is beneath the blastula

2   Decidua capsularis which lies directly over the blastula and separates it from the uterine cavity

3   Decidua vera lines the remainder of the cavity

After successful implantation, the syncytium formed by the outer cell layer of the blastula secretes progesterone, human chorionic gonadotrophin (HCG) and oestrogens

DEVELOPMENT OF THE PLACENTA

1   The trophoblast becomes differentiated into two layers
   a   Outer layer known as the syncytiotrophoblast or syncytium
   b   Inner layer known as the cytotrophoblast or Langhans layer of primitive mesenchyme

2   The syncytium penetrates deep into the endometrium and forms finger-like 'chorionic villi'. Each villus consists of a core of mesoblast cells which start to hollow out to contain fetal blood vessels

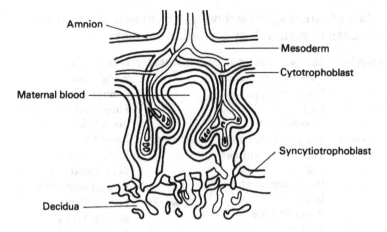

Figure 1.1   *Structure of the placenta*

3 Maternal capillaries erode the syncytium. Maternal blood spills out to form lacunae in the intervillous spaces and exchange of materials occurs with the fetal side of the placental circulation

4 Placenta (Figure 1.1) is fully formed by the 10th week, and at that stage consists of:
 a Cotyledons: these refer to clumps of chorionic villi which are surrounded by:
 b Pools of maternal blood entering at high pressure through spiral arterioles

5 At term the placenta weighs about 500 g and is about 20 cm in diameter

6 Occasionally the placenta has two lobes; if one lobe is small and separate (succenturiate lobe) it may be retained and cause postpartum haemorrhage

DEVELOPMENT OF THE EMBRYO

The term 'embryo' is usually applied to the developing human before 11 weeks post-fertilization; 'fetus' is used after the 12th week post-fertilization.

Basic features of the developing fetus/embryo (refer to textbooks of embryology for fuller details):

4 weeks:	Embryo 1 cm long Yolk sac prominent Eye spots apparent No human resemblance	*20 weeks:*	Length 25 cm Weight 280 g Lanugo all over Fingernails discernible
8 weeks:	Embryo 3 cm long Yolk sac size of hen's egg Head comparatively large Arms and legs present	*24 weeks:*	Length 30 cm Weight 650 g Skin wrinkled and red Eyelids separated
12 weeks:	Embryo length 9 cm Weight 55 g Placenta fully developed Umbilical cord present Fingers and toes present	*28 weeks:*	Length 35 cm Weight 1.1 kg 'Legally viable'; but below 30% survive if born at this stage
		32 weeks:	Length 40 cm Weight 1.6 kg 60% survive if born
16 weeks:	Embryo length 16 cm Weight 150 g Fully sexually differentiated Lanugo appearing; meconium present Heartbeat discernible; fetal movements present	*36 weeks:*	Length 45 cm Weight 2.5 kg Lanugo disappearing Skin becoming less red
		40 weeks; term:	Length 50 cm Weight around 3.5 kg Skin smooth Plentiful subcutaneous fat

FUNCTIONS OF THE PLACENTA

1 Nutrition: Exchange of materials such as glucose and amino acids

2 Respiration: Note that the oxygen tension in efferent blood in the umbilical vein is only about 30% of that in the maternal arterial blood, and normal fetal arterial

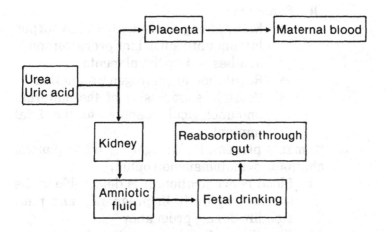

Figure 1.2 *Excretory functions of the placenta*

blood contains as much carbon dioxide as maternal venous blood

3 Excretion: Disposal of waste products, e.g. urea (Figure 1.2)
4 Immunological:
   a At tissue level, 'mixing' of maternal and fetal tissues. It is not known why fetal 'rejection' does not occur
   b Certain maternal antibodies such as immunoglobulin G (IgG) are transferred across the placenta. They provide the fetus with passive immunity
5 Endocrine: The syncytiotrophoblast synthesizes:
   a Human chorionic gonadotrophin (HCG):
      i Blood concentration: Rise to a maximum at 10–11 weeks and then fall, finally disappearing by the first week after birth. Blood concentration is important in the diagnosis of pregnancy and in clinical assessment of a threatened abortion

  ii Functions:
- Maintaining the activity of the corpus luteum until sufficient progesterone is synthesized by the placenta
- Regulation of oestrogen production
- Possible suppression of the maternal immunological reaction to the fetal implant

b Human placental lactogen (HPL) (human chorionic somatomammmotrophin)

  i Blood concentration: It is detectable in the serum very early in pregnancy and rises steadily during pregnancy

  ii Functions: Causes growth of secretory tissue in the breasts and may have an important anabolic effect on mother and fetus

c Oestrogens: The placenta cannot synthesize oestrogens *per se*. It requires other steroid substances as precursors. These are supplied principally by the fetus. Hence the 'fetoplacental unit' is the source of oestrogenic hormones

  i Blood concentration: Increases to a maximum at full term, and is therefore an important means for assessing placental function

  ii Functions: See endocrine section above

d Progesterone:

  i Blood concentration: Rises to a peak at full term

  ii Functions:
- Inhibition of myometrial excitability
- Aids in breast development
- Produces an increase in body temperature

6 Barrier:

 a Protection against harmful substance

b Many harmful substances can pass across the placenta
  i Drugs – thalidomide, warfarin, phenytoin, quinine
  ii Viruses – rubella, cytomegalovirus, herpesvirus
  iii Bacteria – syphilis
  iv Protozoa – toxoplasma

FETAL CIRCULATION

Two umbilical arteries carry blood to the placenta and a single umbilical vein returns blood from the placenta to the portal vein (Figure 1.3). Note the following points about the fetal circulation:

1 Lungs: fetal lungs filled with fluid and are not functional

2 Placenta: this performs functions of respiration, excretion and nutrition

3 Haemodynamics: there is considerable mixing of fetal arterial and venous blood due to:
  a Ductus venosus: blood from the placenta is carried in the umbilical vein. This in turn joins the portal vein but much of this blood proceeds directly to the inferior vena cava via the ductus venosus and thus bypasses the liver
  At birth:
    i The umbilical vein collapses
    ii The ductus venosus becomes a fibrous thread called the ligamentum venosum, so all the blood in the portal vein must now pass through the liver
  b Foramen ovale: this pierces the septum between left and right atria:
    i Before birth: most venous blood entering the right atrium is shunted directly into the left

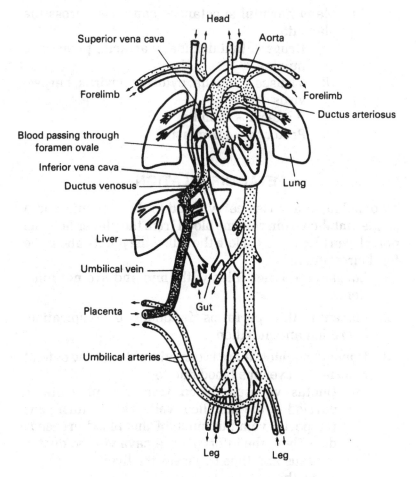

Figure 1.3 *Fetal circulation*

atrium and thence into the systemic circulation
ii At birth: decreased pulmonary resistance
and altered pulmonary pressures close the
flap valve of the foramen ovale, and stop the
diversion of blood.
c Ductus arteriosus: this is a communicating blood

vessel between the pulmonary artery and the aortic arch:

i Before birth: blood from the right ventricle flowing through the pulmonary artery is shunted from the pulmonary circulation into the aorta

ii At birth: decreased pulmonary resistance encourages blood flow to lungs. The increased oxygen saturation of blood causes the smooth muscle of the ductus arteriosus to constrict and the ductus arteriosus closes, to produce a fibrous cord, called the ligamentum arteriosum.

ASSESSMENT OF THE FETUS BEFORE DELIVERY

This is more fully covered in the obstetrics volume of the series. Briefly, the techniques used are:

1 Ultrasound: This may be used to measure fetal biparietal diameter (BPD) and abdominal girth

2 Amniocentesis
   a In early pregnancy this is used for:
      i Detection of genetic abnormalities
      ii Detection of elevated levels of alpha-fetoprotein
   b In late pregnancy this is used for:
      i Assessment of bilirubin levels in suspected or established Rhesus haemolytic disease
      ii Assessment of fetal maturity by measurement of lecithin/sphingomyelin ratio in amniotic fluid

3 Fetal heart rate monitoring: This assesses fetal heart rate and its response to uterine contractions during labour

4 Fetal scalp blood monitoring: This detects fetal blood

pH and lactic acid and monitors fetal acid–base status.

5 Amnioscopy: Is used to examine the colour and consistency of amniotic fluid through intact fetal membranes.

6 Fetal respiratory movements. The fetus shows respiratory movements *in utero*, and these can provide an indication of fetal well-being.

7 Radiography: assessment of fetal gestational age

2

The Delivery Room

PHYSIOLOGICAL ADJUSTMENTS AROUND THE TIME OF BIRTH

Initiation of respiration

This is the primary aim of resuscitation of the newborn (page 33)

1 Before birth, fetal blood–gas exchange occurs in the placenta. Respiratory movements do nevertheless occur in the fetus, and can be used to assess maturation of the fetal nervous system

2 At birth:

  a The trigger to respiration is probably afferent inputs from:

    i Peripheral chemoreceptors in the aortic and carotid bodies

    ii Skin receptors responding to temperature, tactile and sometimes painful contact with the outside world

  b Continued impetus to respiration requires a responsive respiratory centre. This may be impaired by:

    i Administration of sedatives and other drugs such as pethidine to mother during labour

19

ii   Chronic fetal hypoxia during pregnancy
iii Brain injury during delivery

Mechanics of respiration

1   Normal respiration requires a clean and patent airway. This may be impaired by:
    a   Presence of amniotic fluid, blood or meconium in the infant's airway
    b   Abnormality of motor nerves, respiratory muscles or other components of the thoracic cage

2   The first breath requires a large muscular effort to render the lung alveoli patent

3   Subsequent breathing requires less effort in the presence of adequate surfactant. Breathing is impaired in respiratory distress syndrome. See Chapter 7

4   Failure of any of the above steps will result in an acute or chronic hypoxia in the newborn. See page 189

Cardiovascular changes

1   At birth there is an increase in blood flow to the lungs

2   The foramen ovale (see Chapter 1) and ductus arteriosus shunts become closed

3   The circulation now consists of two separate circuits: the pulmonary and systemic circulations
Full circulatory adaptation after birth may be impaired by congenital cardiac abnormalities. See Chapter 8

Changes in blood:
1   The haemoglobin concentration is approximately 18–19 g/dl at birth and this falls to about 12 g/dl. The extra red blood cells are haemolysed and physiological jaundice may result (see page 127)

2 The change from synthesis of fetal haemoglobin (HbF) to adult haemoglobin (HbA) starts to occur *in utero* and is complete by 2 years of age

3 Hypoprothrombinaemia caused by a lack of vitamin K occurs between the first and fifth days after delivery. This may produce haemorrhagic disease of the newborn (see page 141)

Temperature control

1 Before birth: Fetus relies on temperature control mechanisms of mother

2 After birth: Newborn is unable to shiver and depends on:
   a Rapid oxidation and energy production in brown adipose tissue (brown fat)
   b Ultimately – depends on energy content of the diet and surrounding environmental temperature

3 To minimize the energy demand of thermoregulation:
   a Clothe baby in thermally protective materials
   b Maintain an ambient temperature to minimize energy needed to keep core temperature constant

4 Incubators allow close observation and easy access to an infant in a neutral thermal environment. Thermoregulatory problems are common in low birth weight babies (page 51), in the presence of neonatal infection (page 143) and in respiratory distress syndrome (page 93)

Gastrointestinal tract

1 Whereas energy, amino acids, vitamins and certain trace elements are supplied to the fetus via the

placenta, the newborn must derive these nutrients via its diet

2 The gut bacteria that synthesize vitamin K are initially absent and, because vitamin K is needed for the synthesis of prothrombin in the liver, hypoprothrombinaemia may occur

3 Maturation of enzymes: this is only complete after the first few days of life
   a Sugar-splitting enzymes – are easily 'overloaded' in the first week of life
   b Fats: often malabsorption of fats gives problems such as diarrhoea

4 Management of diet:
   a Problems of diet least likely with infant feeding with human breast milk (see page 40)
   b Problems of nutrition may occur in the pre-term infant

Liver function

1 Conjugation of (toxic) bilirubin to (non-toxic) bilirubin diglucuronide by the liver enzyme glucuronyl transferase is not fully developed in the first few days after birth. An increased level of unconjugated bilirubin may cause neonatal jaundice (see page 127); elevated levels of such fat-soluble unconjugated bilirubin may cause kernicterus.

2 Synthesis of serum proteins, and of prothrombin from vitamin K, is submaximal in the first few days of life

3 Liver function may be compromised causing clinical problems, in
   a Pre-term infant (page 52)
   b Hypoxia (page 89)
   c Hypoglycaemia (page 157)
   d Infection (page 143)

Renal function

1 Glomerular filtration rate is lower due to relative underdevelopment of cortical nephrons.

2 Kidney of the newborn is poorly suited to:
  a Excrete a saline load and hypernatraemia may result especially from bottle-feeding
  b Concentrate urine
  c Excrete ammonium compounds and so correct metabolic acidosis – especially in pre-term infants

Immunological system

1 Maternal immunoglobulins: only IgG can cross the placenta and this is in the last trimester. IgG confers a passive immunity to the fetus. Maternal IgG disappears after the first few weeks of life but may confer a relative protection against postnatal virus diseases

2 Fetal immunoglobulins: IgM, IgG and IgE are produced from mid-term onwards by the spleen, but immunoglobulin levels are not appreciable in the absence of an antigenic challenge, for example as caused by an intrauterine infection. The infant is particularly susceptible to infection in the first trimester (see page 144)

3 Newborn immunoglobulins: IgM synthesis increases shortly after birth, but the relative lack of IgM may predispose the newborn to Gram-negative systemic infection. Elevated IgM levels at birth imply intrauterine infection (see page 144)

4 Human breast milk: this contains among other nutrients IgA, lactoferrin, lysozymes and lymphocytes and cells which reduce the incidence of gastrointestinal infection in the newborn

5 The inflammatory response is fully developed before birth. However the neonate is often unable to mount a response effectively at the site of infections. It is therefore susceptible to Gram-positive skin infection (see page 154).

RESUSCITATION OF THE NEWBORN

Anticipation of the infant at risk and preparation of resuscitation equipment are essential prerequisites

Principles of resuscitation

A – Airway management

B – Breathing

C – Circulation

D – Drugs

Possible steps (in ascending order)

1 Clear airways by prompt gentle suction of pharynx, mouth and nostrils (nostrils most important since mouth-breathing only occurs after the neonatal period). Keep neonate warm. Remove vernix and blood etc. from skin to minimize heat loss by evaporation.

2 Place infant on resuscitation table with head slightly downwards. Supply oxygen by mask or intranasal catheter

3 Stimulate movement by drying infant in towel

4 If infant not breathing after 1–2 min:
   a Give 1 mmol/kg sodium bicarbonate intravenously into umbilical vein to correct acidosis
   b If respiratory depression is due to opiates give the opiate antagonist naloxone 0.02 mg/kg preferably intramuscularly

5 If heart rate less than 80/min with no breathing at 1 min despite administered oxygen and stimulation,

consider intubation. If heart rate over 100/min and no breathing, consider intubation after 2 min

6 If circulatory failure occurs administer external cardiac massage

Prognosis:
After resuscitation the asphyxiated infant may encounter many problems, and transfer to a special care baby unit (SCBU) may be necessary. Some of the problems include:

1 Hypothermia

2 Respiratory problems (respiratory distress syndrome, atelectasis, pneumothorax, pneumonia)

3 Hypoglycaemia

4 Depression of central nervous system due to cerebral oedema

5 Hypotension

6 Impaired renal function

7 Haemorrhage due to disseminated intravascular coagulation

Indications for alerting a paediatrician to a delivery

1 Maternal disease
    a Pre-eclampsia and/or eclampsia
    b Diabetes mellitus
    c Hypertension
    d Renal disease
    e Pulmonary disease
    f Cardiac disease
    g Abruptio placentae
    h Placenta praevia

2 Fetal problems
    a Intrauterine growth retardation
    b Rhesus haemolytic disease

    c Evidence of fetal asphyxia
      i Meconium staining
      ii Abnormal fetal heart rate pattern
    d Prematurity or postmaturity

3 Labour and delivery problems
    a Rupture of membranes for over 24 h
    b Abnormal presentation
    c Dystocia
    d Multiple pregnancy
    e Caesarean section

ASSESSMENT OF THE NEWBORN BABY

Aim of assessment

1 Detection of congenital malformations, especially those which may threaten life or need correction later

2 Detection of problems that may have arisen during pregnancy or during delivery, e.g.: haemolytic disease, birth asphyxia, etc.

3 Measurement of parameters of body size

4 Assessment of gestational age

Examination of the newborn

General: Examine baby undressed.
1 Check history of pregnancy and labour and family history

2 Work from head downwards in examination

3 Weight: 3.5 kg at 50th percentile

Head:

Cranial vault:
    a Head circumference: 35 cm at 50th percentile

    b Check size of fontanelles and degree of separation of cranial sutures. The anterior fontanelle is easily palpated but the posterior fontanelle may be closed

    c Check for cephalohaematoma, caput succedaneum and moulding

Face:

    a Check overall facial appearance, including ears for symmetry and position

    b Eyes: inspect for cataract, colobomas, clarity of cornea and subconjunctival haemorrhages and conjunctivitis. Note the angle of the eyes

    c Mouth: check for cleft palate and cleft lip. Teeth are rarely present at birth. Check for sucking reflex

Neck:

    a Examine clavicles to exclude fractures

    b Inspect for sternomastoid 'tumour'

    c Palpate the thyroid gland for enlargement

Thorax:

1 Check for asymmetry and retraction of sternum, ribs or epigastrium.

2 Respiration: Respiratory rate about 40–60 breaths/ min.

3 Cardiovascular: Apex beat normally about 120–160 beats/min; systolic murmurs not uncommon, but should be reviewed later. Check peripheral pulses including femoral pulse

NB: Check for signs of cardiorespiratory problems viz: dyspnoea, indrawing chest wall, cyanosis etc.

Skin:
Look for the following:

Feature	Possible causes
1 Pallor:	**a** Haemorrhage **b** Haemolytic disease **c** Neurological 'shock'
2 Plethora:	**a** Prematurity **b** Polycythaemia **c** Hypo- or hyperthermia
3 Jaundice:	See Chapter 9
4 Cyanosis:	Central cyanosis implies cardio-respiratory disease
5 Skin blemishes:	Haemangiomata, mongolian spot, strawberry naevi

Abdomen:
1 Usually distended and moves with respiration
2 Check umbilical cord for two arteries and one vein, and that it is securely clamped
3 Liver palpable 1–2 cm below costal margin
4 Kidneys usually palpable
5 Bladder should not be palpable after micturition

Perineum:
1 Palpate for hernias
2 Check that anus is patent and in the correct position. Stools: greenish-black meconium for 48 h
3 Males: Check prepuce and descent of both testes into scrotum
   Check for hydrocoele and hypospadias
4 Females: Check for labial fusion and clitoris enlargement. A vaginal discharge is common

Musculoskeletal system:

1 Check spine for evidence of neural tube defects

2 Check limbs for mobility and talipes and anomalies of the digits

3 Examine for congenital dislocation of the hip – Barlow's test (see Chapter 6)

Central nervous system:

1 Observe posture and reflexes

2 Observe behaviour in response to being examined

NB: If normal, reassure mother of normality of her baby

3 Note the presence of the following reflexes
   a Sucking and swallowing reflex
   b Searching reflex – evoked by touching the corner of the baby's mouth
   c Grasp reflex
   d Moro ('embrace' or 'startle') reflex – test by dropping the baby's head from one hand to the other – the baby throws out his arms and then brings them together again
   e Walking reflex

Estimation of gestational age of the newborn

1 Maternal data: Mother's last menstrual period. Data collected during the antenatal period

2 Physical criteria (For further details see Dubowitz et al. (1970) J. Pediat., 77, 1)

3 Neurological criteria:

		Immaturity	Maturity
a	Posture:	Lies flat pelvis held low	Increased flexor tone: high pelvis Knees drawn up under abdomen

Assessment of gestational age: physical criteria (Dubowitz

External sign	0	1
Oedema	Obvious oedema hands and feet; pitting over tibia	No obvious oedema hands and feet; pitting over tibia
Skin texture	Very thin, gelatinous	Thin and smooth
Skin colour (infant not crying)	Dark red	Uniformly pink
Skin opacity (trunk)	Numerous veins and venules clearly seen, especially over abdomen	Veins and tributaries seen
Lanugo (over back)	No lanugo	Abundant; long and thick over whole back
Plantar creases	No skin creases	Faint red marks over anterior half of sole
Nipple formation	Nipple barely visible; no areola	Nipple well defined; areola smooth and flat; diameter <0.75 cm
Breast size	No breast tissue palpable	Breast tissue on one or both sides <0.5 cm diameter
Ear form	Pinna flat and shapeless, little or no incurving of edge	Incurving of part of edge of pinna
Ear firmness	Pinna soft, easily folded, no recoil	Pinna soft, easily folded, slow recoil
Genitalia (male)	Neither testis in scrotum	At least one testis high in scrotum
Genitalia (female) (with hips half abducted)	Labia majora widely separated, labia minora protruding	Labia majora almost cover labia minora

et al., 1970)

	Score	
2	3	4

No oedema

Smooth; medium thickness. Rash or superficial peeling	Slight thickening. Superficial cracking and peeling especially hands and feet	Thick and parchment-like: superficial or deep cracking
Pale pink: variable over body	Pale. Only pink over ears, lips, palms or soles	
A few large vessels clearly seen over abdomen	A few large vessels seen indistinctly over abdomen	No blood vessels seen
Hair thinning especially over lower back	Small amount of lanugo and bald areas	At least half of back devoid of lanugo
Definite red marks over more than anterior half; indentations over less than anterior third	Indentations over more than anterior third	Definite deep indentations over more than anterior third
Areola stippled, edge not raised; diameter <0.75 cm	Areola stippled, edge raised; diameter >0.75 cm	
Breast tissue both sides; one or both 0.5–1.0 cm	Breast tissue both sides; one or both >1 cm	
Partial incurving whole of upper pinna	Well-defined incurving whole of upper pinna	
Cartilage to edge of pinna, but soft in places, ready recoil	Pinna firm, cartilage to edge, instant recoil	
At least one testis right down		
Labia majora completely cover labia minora		

b Reflexes: Appearance of certain reflexes by weeks of gestation

		Present	Absent
		(weeks of gestation)	
i	Reaction of pupils to light	29 +	< 31
ii	Glabella tap (blink on tapping root of nose)	32 +	< 34
iii	Head turning to diffuse light	32 +	doubtful
iv	Traction	33 +	< 36
v	Neck righting	34 +	< 37

3

Care of the Newborn

DELIVERY ROOM MANAGEMENT OF THE NORMAL NEWBORN

1 Maternal history:
   a Maternal age
   b Gravidity and parity
   c Significant maternal illness
   d Maternal medication
   e Obstetric complications
   f Maternal Rh and blood type
   g Time of rupture of membranes
   h Fetal presentation
   i Type of delivery
   j Type of analgesia
   k Fetal monitoring records

2 Suction of mouth, then nose of infant

3 Clamp and cut umbilical cord with infant at perineal level

4 Maintain infant temperature

5 Assess infant's condition and need for resuscitation

6 Assess Apgar scores at 1 and 5 min

7 Brief physical examination with diagnosis of congenital anomalies (see below)

33

8 Estimation of gestational age and comparison with weight

9 Decision on appropriate continuing care
    Infants needing special attention
   a Infants of diabetic mothers
   b Pre-eclamptic or eclamptic mothers
   c Infants small for gestational age
   d Non-elective Caesarean section
   e Infants who weigh more than 4.5 kg
   f Infants of mothers with serious medical problems
   g Infants <37 weeks' gestational age
   h Any other infant judged to require special observation

10 Vitamin K

Observations

Daily:
1 Identification: Use of wrist labels

2 General well-being

3 Rectal temperature using a low-reading thermometer. Normal range 36.5–38°C

4 Weight

5 Stools: passing of meconium for first 2–3 days and stools thereafter

6 Monitor fluid intake and urine output; dextrostix test of urine

7 Check blood glucose using heelpricks within first 48 h

Daily care

1 Hygiene of face and especially eyes

2 Mouth and skin – examined for thrush infection

3 Umbilical cord stump – keep clean and dry and observe for signs of infection

4 Buttocks to be washed and dried each time baby is changed

Feeding

Breast or bottle feeding – see below

Neonatal screening procedures:
1 Dextrostix
2 Serum glucose
3 Haematocrit
4 Bilirubin
5 Blood type, Rhesus and Coombs test
6 Guthrie test

NEONATAL NUTRITION

Energy requirements

1 Caloric requirements: Between 100 and 120 kcal kg^{-1} day^{-1}. Since the calorific value of human milk is around 70 kcal/100 ml, this corresponds to a milk intake of around 160–180 ml kg^{-1} day^{-1}. The normal baby can adjust this volume intake according to the caloric content of the milk. The caloric requirement is substantially higher in pre-term infants due to the following factors:
  a Increased caloric demand due to increased requirement for growth and temperature control
  b Increased faecal caloric loss
The requirement may then rise to 140–160 kcal kg^{-1} day^{-1}

2 Utilization of energy in a normal neonate

$$(kcal\,kg^{-1}\,day^{-1})$$

  a Intake   150

  b Utilization:

    i Resting metabolism   50–60

    ii Growth   20–30

    iii Activity   15–20

    iv Faecal loss   10–12

    v Specific dynamic action of food   8–10

3 Fat supply: Milk fat is mainly triglyceride. Around 60% of human milk is in the form of palmitic or oleic acids. Newborn babies are able to absorb 80–90% of their intake of human milk, but only 60–70% if fed on cow's milk. This is because of the higher unsaturated fat content of human milk. Fat absorption is impaired in low-birth weight babies, probably due to a deficiency of pancreatic lipase and bile salts

4 Carbohydrate supply: This is present as lactose in both human (70 g/l) and cows' (50 g/l) milk. It is broken down into glucose and galactose by the action of hydrolytic enzymes

Protein

1 Amount:

  a Normal babies: Require around 2 g kg^{-1} day^{-1}, and most of the protein is used for growth. This corresponds to a milk intake of 180 ml kg^{-1} day^{-1}. Unmodified cows' milk contains a higher level of around 3 g/100 ml, than human milk (1–1.5 g/100 ml). This excess uptake of protein may cause abnormal blood urea levels, and for this reason modified preparations should be used in preference to cows' milk if breast feeding is not possible

b Premature babies: The precise requirement is uncertain, but may be around $4 \text{ g kg}^{-1} \text{ day}^{-1}$. Intakes of below $2 \text{ g kg}^{-1} \text{ day}^{-1}$ result in poor growth and failure to thrive, but intakes of over $5 \text{ g kg}^{-1} \text{ day}^{-1}$ may result in acidosis and elevated levels of blood urea

2 Type of protein:
   a Premature neonates are especially deficient in the following metabolic pathways:
      i Metabolism of methionine to cysteine
      ii Metabolism of phenylalanine to tyrosine and homogentisic acid
      These provide another problem in relation to feeding with cows' milk because this has high levels of phenylalanine and tyrosine, and will lead to elevation of the plasma levels of these amino acids. In addition, cows' milk is deficient in cysteine, an essential amino acid. These problems do not occur with human milk
   b Cows' milk contains a large amount of casein protein in relation to whey protein, whereas the opposite is true for human milk. The casein forms curds in the gastrointestinal tract, and this may impair protein absorption

Minerals

The quantitative requirements of trace elements have not been defined. Around 70% of their body content is transferred from mother to the neonate in the third trimester. In consequence, the pre-term baby is relatively deprived of mineral deposition

1 Monovalent ions: sodium, potassium, chloride: The approximate requirements are:

Na^+	$2-4 \text{ mmol kg}^{-1} \text{ day}^{-1}$
K^+	$1-3 \text{ mmol kg}^{-1} \text{ day}^{-1}$
Cl^-	$2-4 \text{ mmol kg}^{-1} \text{ day}^{-1}$

However, the following points should be noted:

a   Most formulas do supply enough of these ions to meet requirements, even in the premature

b   The sodium content of cows' milk is considerably higher (600 mg/l) than in human milk (150 mg/l), and this may predispose to hypernatraemic dehydration (Chapter 16), especially if made up to too high a concentration, or if there is a condition that results in dehydration. However particular preparations of milk are obtainable which have a more physiological sodium concentration

2   Calcium:

a   Requirements may be high in the neonatal period so that calcification keeps pace with the formation of new bone matrix. Human milk contains 320–340 mg/l calcium, and most preparations may contain up to 1 g/l of calcium. However, absorption of calcium may be variable, and loss of the calcium in the stools correlates closely with its lipid content

b   In premature infants, calcium requirements may be over 200 mg kg^{-1} day^{-1}, and rates of absorption may be further compromised resulting in osteoporotic bone changes and poor rates of growth. Calcium supplementation is therefore employed in some centres for such infants

3   Phosphate: The daily requirement of phosphate is unknown; however, probably the optimum ratio of calcium to phosphate approaches that in human milk. Furthermore, the newborn baby is deficient in its ability to excrete large quantities of phosphate, and the elevated phosphate level that may result with feeding with cows' milk may predispose to hypocalcaemic tetany of the newborn

4 Iron:
  a In the normal newborn, the total body iron is around 270–310 mg, but most of this is present as the red cell mass. In the first 2 months of life this red cell mass decreases, and the iron so liberated is stored. After this, erythropoiesis becomes active, and the stored iron is used up. Neither human nor cows' milk is rich in iron
  b Premature babies are born with a smaller red cell mass. They may therefore require iron supplementation after 8 weeks, to avoid a hypochromic anaemia

Vitamins

1 Vitamin K: Both premature and full-term infants at birth should be treated with 0.5–1.0 mg vitamin K, intramuscularly. This is to avoid haemorrhagic disease of the newborn. Usually only one dose is required, as the establishment of normal intestinal flora results in an adequate supply of vitamin K. However, where the gut flora is not adequately established, e.g. during antibiotic therapy, further doses of vitamin K may be indicated

2 Vitamin A: The daily requirement of vitamin A is around 500 iu. One pint of human milk contains between 500 and 1000 iu, and supplemented cows' milk may contain up to 1700 iu/500 ml. Hence the infant is likely to derive all its requirement for this vitamin without difficulty

3 Vitamin C: The infant may require up to 20 mg/day. However, human milk is rich in this vitamin, but cows' milk (unless modified or fortified') is a poor source, and under the latter condition some vitamin C supplements may be desirable

4   Vitamin D: The recommended requirement is around 400 iu/day, and so supplementation is required from around a month after birth. This is especially important for premature babies, who may need 800–1200 iu/day

5   Folic acid: Around 50 μg are needed per day; the amount of folic acid in human milk is around 50 μg/l, and that in supplemented cows' milk is around 20 μg/l. Hence a daily dose of around 50 μg/day from birth of folic acid is desirable to protect against megaloblastic anaemia

6   Vitamin E: The newborn requires between 5 and 25 iu per day; the exact figure is uncertain. Human milk contains only 5 iu/l, and cows' milk 3 iu/l of vitamin E. Hence, in order to prevent a deficiency, daily supplementation with around 5–25 iu of tocopherol acetate may be desirable in premature babies. Vitamin E deficiency causes oedema, haemolytic anaemia and thrombocytosis

BREAST-FEEDING

During the first few days the infant will receive colostrum, a high-calorie, high-protein 'milk' rich in antibodies, lymphocytes, macrophages and other essential nutrients. Milk does not 'come in' until 48–72 h postpartum. Unless it is contraindicated (see below) the mother should be encouraged to breast-feed.

Antenatal preparation for breast-feeding

1   Patient should regularly massage breasts towards the nipple to expel colostrum. Removal of colostrum helps to develop the duct system and prevents it becoming blocked

2   Adequate hygiene of nipples

3 Antenatal education on advantages and method of breast-feeding

4 If nipples are inverted a nipple shield should be worn under a brassiere

Establishment of breast-feeding

Requirements for success:
1 Milk secretion by alveoli

2 Operative milk ejection reflex

3 Mother must be motivated to feed

4 Good diet and rest for nursing mother

Points to establish:
1 Both mother and baby to be made comfortable during breast-feeding

2 The sooner the baby is put to the breast, the more successful is lactation

3 Mother needs to be shown fully the technique of breast-feeding

4 Once breast-feeding is established, feeding to be 'on demand'

5 Breast-feeding stopped as late as possible

Chemical composition of milks

| | Human | Cow | Commercial milks | |
			Unmodified	Modified
Lipid (g/dl)	3.8	3.7	3.3	3.0–3.5
Protein (g/dl)	1.0–1.2	3.3	3.3	1.5–1.8
Carbohydrate (g/dl)	7.0	4.8	6.7–7.0	7.0
Sodium (mmol/l)	10	58	50–56	15–33
Phosphate (mg/dl)	15	96	88–95	33–50
Iron (mg/dl)	0.15	0.10	1.0	1.0

Advantages of breast-feeding

The composition of breast milk is ideal for normal growth and development – nature knows best!
1 To the infant:
  a Breast milk is more physiological in composition. In addition to essential nutrients, breast milk contains many anti-infectious agents including:
    i Leukocytes
    ii Macrophages
    iii Immunoglobulins A and G (IgA, IgG)
    iv Lysozyme
    v Lactoferrin
    vi Complement
  b Lower incidence in the infant of:
    i Gastroenteritis and other infections
    ii Obesity
    iii Electrolyte problems, e.g. hypernatraemic dehydration
    iv Cot deaths (but aetiology of this is not clear, see below)
    v Neonatal tetany, due to hypocalcaemia secondary to hyperphosphataemia from bottle-feeding preparations
    vi Later childhood illnesses, e.g. asthma
    vii Intussusception
2 To the mother:
  a Enhanced maternal–infant bonding
  b Maternal satisfaction
  c Economy and requires no preparation
  d Increased fat mobilization during lactation helps mother to return to her normal pre-pregnancy weight

Problems of breast-feeding

1 Infant receives no calories for first 48 h postnatally

2   Initial discomfort to mother

3   Inadequate iron after 3 months

4   Inadequate supply of milk

5   Passage of drugs into breast milk

6   Not a good contraceptive

Factors influencing passage of a drug into breast milk:
1   Ionization: The plasma pH of 7.4 is higher than milk, pH 6.8. Hence basic drugs are more concentrated in milk than acidic drugs

2   Lipid solubility: Lipid-soluble drugs will pass easily into breast milk

3   Protein binding: Drugs highly bound to plasma proteins will only appear sparingly in breast milk

4   Molecular size: Water-soluble small molecules are more likely to enter breast milk

Drugs known to cause adverse effects in breast-fed babies (see also Appendix):
1   Alcohol: Causes sedation

2   Ampicillin: Candidiasis, diarrhoea

3   Sulphonamides: Neonatal jaundice

4   Benzodiazepines: Lethargy, weight loss

5   Barbiturates: Drowsiness

6   Lithium: Hypotonia; goitre

7   Ergot alkaloids: Ergotism

8   Tetracycline: Discoloration of teeth

9   Antithyrotoxic drugs: hypothyroidism

Breast engorgement

In some women, particularly primiparae, milk 'comes in' too quickly and breast engorgement occurs

Cause: Failure of the milk-ejection reflex producing engorgement of breasts with milk

Clinical features:
1 Breasts turgid and tender
2 Individual lobules can be palpated as 'knotted lumps'
3 Skin becomes tense and hot
4 Feeding is often agonizing

Treatment:
1 Continue breast-feeding, if possible, to promote milk-ejection reflex
2 Cold packs
3 Analgesia
4 Oestrogens – stilboestrol 5–15 mg, repeated at 4 hourly intervals if necessary; this has now been superseded by bromocriptine
5 Bromocriptine 2.5 mg (1st day), then 2.5 mg b.d. for 14 days

Complications:
1 Cracked nipple
2 Breast abscess

Acute mastitis and breast abscess

Cause: Infection from skin of baby, often staphylococcal

Clinical features:
1 Pyrexia and chills
2 Hard and red, tender breasts

Treatment:
1 Analgesia with antibiotics, e.g. flucloxacillin

2 Continue breast-feeding if possible

3 Drain abscess if present

Suppression of lactation

Indications:

1 Mother wishing to bottle-feed infant

2 Where breast-feeding is stopped because of cracked nipples, acute mastitis, or breast abscess

Method:

1 Natural method – mother encouraged to wear a firm brassiere

2 Use of drugs: bromocriptine (2.5 mg (first day), then 2.5 mg b.d. for 14 days) inhibits the secretion of prolactin from the anterior pituitary

Contraindications to breast-feeding:

1 Mother finds idea of breast-feeding repulsive

2 Unmarried mother planning to have her baby adopted

3 Maternal medical conditions:
   a Severe cardiac conditions
   b Pulmonary tuberculosis
   c Unstable diabetes mellitus

4 Maternal psychiatric disorders

5 Congenital malformations of the baby:
   a Cleft lip and palate in some cases
   b Cardiac abnormalities in some severe cases

Advantages of bottle feeding

1 Possible to determine how much the baby takes without test-weighing

2 Smaller risk of iron deficiency

3   Many drugs are excreted into breast milk (e.g. alcohol, nicotine, caffeine, diazepam, salicylates)

4   More convenient to some

Disadvantages of bottle feeding

1   Reduced calcium availability. Fat is not well absorbed and calcium combines with free fatty acids. Hypocalcaemia results and convulsions may occur in the first week of life

2   Risk of infection from dirty preparation and administration of feed

3   Gastroenteritis is more common

4   Problem of too much or too little food

5   Exposure to allergens

THE MOTHER–BABY RELATIONSHIP

Development of maternal attachment to infant

1   Mother's emotional attachment to baby begins from early pregnancy. In the case of death of fetus or newborn, the mother will experience a period of mourning

2   At birth, mother's initial concern is often for health and normality of baby. Mother then develops full attachment to infant by prolonged closeness to baby

3   Hence, where possible, prolonged separation of mother and child or rigidity of postnatal regime should be avoided

Management of mother of a sick infant

In the delivery room:
1   Prompt survey of the seriousness of the condition and decisions about immediate treatment

2 Indicate to the mother there is a problem and give an indication of the type of trouble

3 If the baby is likely to die, or requires removal from the room, mother should be informed and assured of news of progress. Mother should not be prevented from seeing a sick or deformed infant

In the special care baby unit:
1 The mother's comfort and access to seeing her baby remain important

2 Mother should be prepared for her baby's appearance and the equipment used in the baby unit

3 There should always be available advice from medical and nursing staff

Subsequent reactions: Parents may go through a period of shock, with feelings of disappointment and guilt, and will require continued support and understanding over the succeeding weeks.

DISCHARGE EXAMINATION

1 Central nervous system: Activity, fullness of fontanelle

2 Heart – development of murmur or signs of cardiac failure

3 Skin – jaundice

4 Abdomen – masses or distension

5 Stools and urine output

6 Cord – infection

7 Feeding – breast or bottle

8 Maternal ability to provide adequate care

9 Follow-up – if necessary

DEVELOPMENTAL SCREENING AFTER DISCHARGE

1 Indications:
  a Infants found to have problems around the peri-natal period; e.g. a pre-term infant should be examined 6 weeks after the expected date of delivery (EDD)
  b Total population screening: assessment should be performed:
     i   Within 24 h of birth (see above)
     ii At 6 weeks
     iii At 8 months
     iv At 18 months
     The aim of this primary examination is to detect possible abnormalities that may require further paediatric attention

2 General examination at 6 weeks:
  a Alertness and responsiveness
  b Interest in surroundings
  c Ability to concentrate

3 Visual development:
  a Infant should be able to fixate on, and follow, the examiner's face
  b Infant should be observed for any squint that may be developing

4 Motor function:
  a Infant placed prone eventually briefly raises his head
  b Infant lifted in the prone position: head should rise level with trunk

5 Other points:
  a Testes: Descent in males
  b Hips: For congenital dislocation. This is best detected at the first examination within 24 h
  c Cardiovascular system: Heart sounds; femoral pulses

Features of non-accidental injury (battered baby syndrome)

1 Child shows features of neglect, or failure to thrive

2 Delay between alleged accident and parents seeking medical help

3 Previous history of suspicious injury

4 Explanation of the injury is unsatisfactory, or too plausible

5 Injuries include (initially):
     a Burns
     b Abrasions
     c Injuries to the mouth
     d Bruises
     e Subconjunctival haemorrhages
     f Fractures
     g Head injuries

4

Gestational Age and Birth Weight

Definition of terms

1 Low birth weight ('premature'): Refers to a weight of 2.5 kg (5½ lb) or less at birth

2 Pre-term baby has a gestation period of less than 37 weeks

3 Full-term baby has a gestation period of 38–41 weeks

4 Post-mature baby has a gestation period of more than 42 weeks

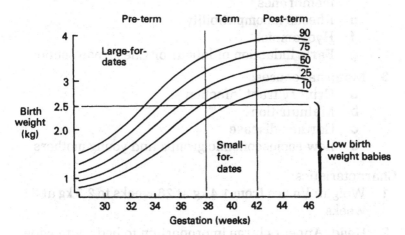

Figure 4.1 *Classification of infants by birth weight and gestation*

51

5 Small-for-dates baby has a birth weight below the 10th percentile for his gestational age (see Figure 4.1)

6 Large-for-dates baby has a birth weight above the 90th percentile for his gestational age (see Figure 4.1)

A low birth weight infant may be either a pre-term or a small-for-dates baby

THE PRE-TERM BABY

Incidence: About 7% of live births

Aetiology:
1 Unknown (about 50%)
2 Obstetric causes:
   a Antepartum haemorrhage from placenta praevia or abruptio placentae
   b Multiple pregnancy
   c Congenital abnormalities
   d Incompetent cervix and premature rupture of membranes
   e Rhesus incompatibility
   f Hydramnios
   g Early induction of labour or Caesarean section

3 Maternal causes:
   a Urinary tract infection
   b Malnutrition
   c Cardiac disease
   d Low socioeconomic groups and young mothers

Characteristics:
1 Weight: Varies from 1.4 kg at 28 weeks to 2.5 kg at 34 weeks
2 Head: Appears large in proportion to body with wide sutures and fontanelles
3 Skin: Thin and translucent with scanty subcutaneous tissue

4 Chest: Appears short compared with abdomen with a prominent rib cage

5 Abdomen: Peristalsis may be visible

6 Genitalia: Undescended testis in male. In female labia minora not covered by labia majora

7 Reflexes: Absent or poorly developed

Problems of the pre-term baby

1 Feeding problems due to:
   a Poorly developed rooting, sucking and swallowing reflexes
   b Ease of regurgitation (small stomach and poor tone of oesophageal sphincter mechanism)
   c Large calorie requirements (best given by nasogastric tube)

2 Jaundice frequent because of immaturity of conjugating enzymes in liver

3 Respiratory distress syndrome – alveolar collapse and atelectasis

4 Breathing often irregular in rhythm and depth

5 Infection owing to poor passive immunity – decreased placental transfer of immunoglobulins – the incidence of meningitis and sepsis is four times greater than in full-term newborns

6 Poor temperature control – large body area to body mass, and lack of subcutaneous fat. Susceptible to hypothermia and hyperthermia

7 Brain damage – hypoxia

8 Anaemia and general vitamin deficiency

9 Bleeding tendency – because of limited ability of liver to utilize vitamin K

10 Susceptibility to hyperoxia – retrolental fibroplasia (see Chapter 7)

11 Poor tolerance to drugs

12 Impaired mother–infant bonding

THE SMALL-FOR-DATES BABY (GROWTH-RETARDED OR LIGHT-FOR-DATES BABY)

Incidence: In UK about 5% all live births

Aetiology:
1 Genetic and congenital factors – chromosomal abnormalities, e.g. trisomy 21, 13, 18
2 Placental insufficiency – as a result of maternal:
   a Malnutrition
   b Hypertension
   c Pre-eclampsia
   d Heart disease
   e Renal disease
   f Severe diabetes mellitus
   g Multiple pregnancy
   h Threatened abortion
   i Excessive smoking
   j Chronic alcoholism
3 Intrauterine infection:
   a Cytomegalovirus
   b Toxoplasmosis
   c Rubella
   d Herpes simplex
   e Syphilis
4 No obvious cause

Problems of the small-for-dates baby:
1 Intrauterine:
   a Chronic hypoxia – signs of fetal distress may have presented during labour

   b Intrauterine death – about 5–10 times greater than for fully developed fetus

2 Intrapartum:
   a Acute or chronic hypoxia leading to death (see Chapter 7)
   b Meconium aspiration (see Chapter 7)

3 Postpartum:
   a Hypoglycaemia – due to inadequate stores of glucose – in first 12 h
   b Hypocalcaemia
   c Temperature instability
   d Pulmonary haemorrhage
   e Hyperviscosity of blood causing thrombosis and cardiac failure

Comparison of pre-term baby and small-for-dates baby

	Problem	Pre-term baby	Small-for-dates baby
1	Classification	Born before 37th week of pregnancy	Weight below 10th percentile for gestational age
2	Intrapartum hypoxia and death	Uncommon	Common
3	Neonatal mortality	High	Low
4	Lung problems	Respiratory distress syndrome	Meconium aspiration
5	Hypoglycaemia and hypocalcaemia	Uncommon	Common
6	Skin	Reddish pink. Lanugo present	Dry, wrinkled and scaly
7	Activity	Minimal; lies in 'frog' attitude	Active; takes flexed posture
8	Reflexes and muscle tone	Poor to fair	Fair to good
9	Later growth	Normal	Often short stature

MANAGEMENT OF THE LOW BIRTH WEIGHT INFANT

1 Prevention of pre-term and light-for-dates deliveries:
   a Improved socioeconomic conditions
   b Regular and careful antenatal care
   c Obstetric care

2 After delivery:
   a Adequate resuscitation as necessary at birth
   b Control of temperature of the neonate
   c Consider admission to special care baby unit especially if:
      i   Infant is 2 kg or less
      ii   Evidence of respiratory difficulty
      iii Evidence of defective thermoregulatory mechanisms

3 Perinatal care:
   a Attention to importance of allowing mother–baby relationship to develop, especially in special care baby units
   b Observations:
      i   Temperature, including temperature of incubator, checked at half-hourly to hourly intervals
      ii   Colour – pallor, cyanosis or jaundice
      iii   Respiration (respiratory movements are monitored continuously by the apnoea alarm mattress)
      iv   Heart rate; blood pressure
      v   Activity
      vi   Passage of urine and meconium
      vii   Condition of umbilical cord
      viii Abnormal signs – including convulsions
   c Maintenance of body temperature
      i   Avoid unnecessary exposure
      ii Nurse in incubator if necessary; heat shield; 'baby therm'

d Prevention of infection:
   i Isolation facilities
   ii Hand-washing by staff
   iii Use of gowns, masks and separate shoes in some units
e Feeding:
   i Early bottle-feeding advised to prevent hypoglycaemia, dehydration and jaundice
   ii Breast- or bottle-feeding if sucking and cough reflexes are present
   iii Otherwise if infant unable to suck may have to consider intragastric or jejunal tube feeding. This can be intermittent (every 3 h) or continuous for infants particularly at risk. No baby with respiratory problems should be orally fed until considered 'stable', but even then may not tolerate oral feeds and therefore may need hourly tube-feeding

4 Preparations for discharge:
  a Education of mother in care of infant
  b Mother is encouraged to get used to handling infant
  c Provision of follow-up facilities to assess and assist in progress

Development of low birth weight infants

The majority of infants who survive develop normally. Specialised baby care units (SCBUs) have survival rates up to and over 80%

Physical and intellectual development:
1 Infants born 6 weeks or less before term have much the same development as full-term infants

2 Infants born between 30 and 34 weeks have a less favourable prognosis

3 Infants born before 30 weeks have an increased incidence of neurological impairment

Prognosis

Pre-term baby:
1 Prospects for survival are directly related to birth weight

2 Short term: Overall mortality statistics for pre-term infants born after the 28th week are:
  a 62% of deaths occur in first 24 h
  b 90% of deaths occur over first week
  c 100% of deaths occur over first 6 weeks
  i.e. baby's prospects become brighter as the baby successively survives the first day, week and 6 weeks of life. However, there is a higher incidence of sudden infant death syndrome (cot death) (see Chapter 14)

3 Long term: With neonatal intensive care, baby may continue to develop normally after birth as long as nutritional and nursing requirements are met, but this point awaits fuller assessment.

Small-for-dates baby:
1 Subsequent physical growth may also be affected, depending on the cause of the slow growth

2 Complications may also arise if hypoglycaemia is not treated – may lead to mental retardation, epilepsy and spasticity

Indications for referral to special care baby unit (SCBU)

1 Absolute indications:
  a Birth weight below 1.5 kg
  b Below 32 weeks gestation
  c Respiratory difficulty and/or apnoea
  d Suspected sepsis and/or meningitis

e Convulsions
f Central cyanosis
g Suspected congenital cardiac disease
h Evidence of severe haemolytic disease of the neonate

2 Relative indications:
a Birth weight below 2 kg
b Below 34 weeks gestation
c History of intrauterine growth impairment
d Meconium aspiration
e Infants that required prolonged resuscitation after birth
f Severe congenital abnormality for assessment
g Severe jaundice requiring exchange transfusion

Information required before transfer to SCBU:

1 Mother's name, age, address and telephone number

2 Mother's blood group and reports of antibody testing

3 Date of last menstrual period and expected date of delivery

4 Mother's previous obstetric history

5 5–10 ml of mother's blood (clotted)

6 If Rhesus or other blood-group incompatibility is suspected take 5–10 ml of blood from placental end of umbilical cord

5

Congenital Abnormalities

Probably about half of all conceptions are aborted, and it is thought that the majority of these are associated with congenital abnormalities. Congenital anomalies account for about 10% of neonatal deaths. A major anomaly is present at birth in about 3% of all newborns. There is considerable geographical and racial variation; a good example is anencephaly which has an incidence of 1 in 175 births in Ireland and 1 in 1000 births in Australia.

Aetiology of congenital abnormalities

1 Hereditary genetic defects – responsible for many single malformations as well as syndromes

2 Chromosomal aberrations, which may be familial

3 Defects of uncertain cause such as those due to infections, drugs, irradiation and hypoxia

Hereditary genetic defects

These by definition are familial and there are several types:

1 Autosomal dominant traits: These are manifest in the heterozygous state and the statistical risk of recur-

rence is 50%; that is there is a 50% chance of each subsequent child being similarly affected. Some examples include:

a Marfan's syndrome
b Achondroplasia
c Neurofibromatosis (Von Recklinghausen's disease)
d Huntington's chorea
e Polyposis coli

2 Autosomal recessive traits: These are manifest only with the gene in the homozygous state. The risk to siblings where both parents carry the affected gene is:

a 25% chance of being affected (has abnormal genes)
b 50% chance of being carriers (one normal, one abnormal gene)
c 25% chance of being unaffected (has normal genes)

Some examples are:

i Cystic fibrosis
ii Phenylketonuria
iii Alkaptonuria
iv Wilson's disease
v Galactosaemia
vi Adrenogenital syndrome

3 Autosomal co-dominant traits: In these, the products of both alleles are recognizable; for example: The abnormal haemoglobins, e.g. thalassaemia, sickle cell anaemia

4 Dominant X-linked traits: Affected males will transmit such traits to their daughters but not to their sons; for example:

a Vitamin D-resistant rickets
b Glucose-6-phosphate dehydrogenase deficiency

5 Recessive X-linked traits: In these only males are phenotypically affected but the genotype is transmitted by females; for example:
  a Haemophilia – deficiency in clotting factor VIII
  b Christmas disease – inability to synthesize clotting factor IX

Chromosome aberrations

In simple terms, chromosomal anomalies may be caused by:

1 Non-disjunction. This is the abnormal segregation of chromosomes during cell division, resulting in two chromosome members of the same pair being incorporated in one daughter nucleus. Meiotic non-disjunction involves cells of the germ plasm, and is commoner with high maternal age.

2 Translocation. This is the transfer of a chromosomal segment of one chromosome onto a non-homologous chromosome, resulting in structural chromosomal aberrations. In translocation there is a normal chromosomal complement

3 Mosaicism. This involves the unequal distribution of chromosomes during cell division after fertilisation – mitotic non-disjunction

Examples of chromosomal aberrations are:
  a Down's syndrome (trisomy 21)
  b Edward's syndrome (trisomy 18)
  c Patau's syndrome (trisomy 13)
  d Klinefelter's syndrome (XXY)
  e Turner's syndrome (XO)
  They are discussed in further detail below.

Occurrence of chromosomal abnormalities:
1 Overall: Approximately 0.5–0.6% of the total population of newborn babies have major chromosomal abnormalities

2 Autosomal abnormalities:
  a Abnormalities in chromosomal number: 0.1–0.2% births
  b Abnormalities in chromosomal structure: 0.2–0.3% births
  The commonest autosomal abnormality is Down's syndrome (trisomy 21). Other autosomal abnormalities are rare because they are more likely to be lethal than sex chromosomal abnormalities
3 Sex chromosomal abnormalities: 0.2–0.3% of births. Examples are shown in the table below:

	Nuclear sex chromosomes (buccal smear)	Sex chromosomal pattern as determined by 'squash' preparation	Total number of chromosomes
1 Normal female	+ ve	XX	46
2 Normal male	– ve	XY	46
3 Turner's syndrome	– ve	XO	45
4 Klinefelter's syndrome	+ ve	XXY	47
5 'Superfemale'	+ ve	XXX	47

Clinical importance of the sex chromosomes

1 The X chromosomes:
  a Two X chromosomes are needed for differentiation of the primitive gonads into normal ovaries
  b Genes responsible for carriage of colour-blindness and haemophilia occur on the X chromosome
  c Genes that determine height are located on the X chromosomes. Thus a feature of Turner's syndrome (XO) is short stature (see below)
  d An excess complement of X chromosomes occurs in 'superfemales' (XXX, XXXX,) and Klinefelter's syndrome (XXY) (see below)

2 The Y chromosome:
   a Contains a strong determinant for the male phenotype. Thus a phenotypic male occurs in Klinefelter's syndrome (XXY)
   b Is needed for the development of a functioning testis

Investigation of sex chromosomal abnormalities

1 Buccal smear cytology: This test is based on recognition of the sex chromatin (Barr) body in the cell nucleus adjacent to the nuclear membrane. The Barr body is present in around 70% of nuclei in genetic females and in less than 4% of males. It may be a coiled, temporarily inactivated, X chromosome in the nucleus
2 The 'squash' preparation: This is made by adding colchicine to arrest the cell division of cultured cells at a stage when the nuclei are scattered. The cells are then squashed on a slide in hypotonic salt solutions and examined under magnification

Down's syndrome (Trisomy 21)

First described in 1866 by Down

Incidence:
1 1 in 600 live births
2 2 in 100 live births in mothers over 40
   Paternal age is not related to the condition

Aetiology: majority of subjects have an extra chromosome in the G(21) group. This arises in three ways:
1 Non-disjunction (94%)
2 Translocation (3%)
3 Mosaicism (3%)

A small percentage of subjects have 46 chromosomes with translocation. Trisomy 21 and translocation are clinically indistinguishable

Clinical features:
1 General: Small-for-dates, hypotonia, hyperflexible joints. Happy docile children
2 Head: Rounded and relatively short from front to back:
  a Flat facies
  b Small nose with low bridge
  c Epicanthic folds with upward slant (mongoloid) of eyes
  d Strabismus
  e Speckling of iris (Brushfield's spots)
  f Protruding tongue often fissured ('scrotal' tongue)
3 Short thick neck
4 Transverse single palmar crease (Simian crease); short stubby hands
5 Wide space and plantar crease between first and second toes
6 Mental defect
7 High incidence (about 40%) of congenital cardiac abnormalities
8 Cataracts, duodenal atresia, Hirschsprung's disease and leukaemia are also relatively common

Diagnosis:
1 Clinical features
2 Chromosomal analysis

Management:
1 Parents must be told of diagnosis and offered support
2 Retardation in achieving milestones – mother needs to help child feed, dress, and toilet-train

3 Older child needs special day-school

4 Medical problems are frequent for, e.g., intercurrent respiratory infections

Prognosis: If child survives the neonatal period and has no associated abnormalities then life-expectancy is not much reduced but there is an increased incidence of acute myeloid leukaemia. Behavioural and emotional problems may appear in later life. Not all Down's children are friendly and good-natured.

Genetic counselling: About 2% of neonates are born with a congenital defect. It is therefore necessary for the parents to be informed about the problems of the affected child so that it can be accepted into the family. It will also be necessary to provide advice concerning the chance of a similar defect occurring at the next pregnancy and what steps, if any, can be taken to avoid this risk:

1 Make an accurate diagnosis of the disease

2 Consider:
   a The natural history and prognosis of the disease
   b The risk of the disease transmitting to the next generation
   c Available alternatives to bearing affected children

3 Consider pre-natal diagnosis at around the sixteenth week of pregnancy, as appropriate, by amniocentesis in future pregnancies

NB: Many congenital abnormalities do not follow classical Mendelian inheritance. It may then be necessary to use empirical risk figures

Trisomy 18 syndrome (Edward's syndrome)

Incidence: 1 in about 2000 births

Aetiology: Subjects have an extra chromosome 18. Infants

are normally small for gestational age. Older maternal age is a factor.

Clinical features:
1 Growth failure, mental retardation
2 Open skull sutures and wide fontanelles at birth
3 Protruding occiput, with retroflexion of head
4 High arched eyebrows
5 Low-set deformed ears
6 Micrognathia
7 Flexion deformities of fingers
8 Ventricular septal defect and patent ductus arteriosus
9 Meckel's diverticulum
10 Short sternum
11 Horseshoe kidney
12 Abduction deformity of hips, muscular hypertonus, pes equinovarus
13 Prominent external genitalia with absence of labia majora

Diagnosis:
1 Clinical manifestations
2 Chromosome studies – 47 chromosomes with extra 18 chromosome or an occasional mosaicism.

Management:
1 Over 70% die within 3 months
2 Genetic counselling and family support

Trisomy 13 (D trisomy or Patau's syndrome)

Incidence: 1 in 4000–5000 births

Aetiology: Subjects have an extra chromosome 13 in the D group. Infants normally small for gestational age. Older maternal age is a factor

Clinical features:
1 Growth failure, mental retardation
2 Microcephaly
3 Cleft lip and palate, low-set and deformed ears, deafness, small eyes, with colobomata
4 Polydactyly, flexion deformities of fingers, deformed finger nails, Simian crease
5 Atrial septal defect and ventricular septal defect, dextrocardia; patent ductus arteriosus
6 Kidney cysts, double ureter
7 Umbilical hernia
8 Cryptorchidism

Diagnosis:
1 Clinical manifestations
2 Chromosome studies show an extra chromosome 13 or an occasional mosaicism
3 Increased segmentation of polymorphonuclear granulocytes. Hook-like nucleus

Management:
1 Over 75% die within 3 months
2 Genetic counselling and family support

Turner's syndrome

Disorder of phenotypic females. Chromosome studies show 45 chromosomes although variants and mosaics do exist. There is an association with auto-immune thyroid disease

Clinical features:
1   Small stature
2   'Sphinx' face
3   'Carp' mouth
4   Webbed neck
5   Shield-shaped thorax
6   Coarctation of the aorta
7   Widely spaced nipples
8   Cubitus valgus (increased carrying angle of the upper limb)
9   Poor breast development
10 Short fourth metacarpal
11 Fingernail hypoplasia
12 Lymphoedema at birth
13 Sterile gonads (rudimentary ovaries – contain no follicles)
14 Primary amenorrhoea and infertility
15 Multiple pigmented naevi
16 Kidney and ureteric deformities

Diagnosis:
1   Clinical manifestation
2   Chromosome analysis – most cases are 45 XO although variants and mosaics do occur
3   Elevated serum FSH and LH
4   Urinary gonadotrophin elevated, urinary oestrogens, and 17α-ketosteroids reduced.

Management:
1   Counselling
2   Oestrogen and progesterone therapy to initiate feminization. Treatment should start at 12–13 years of age

Klinefelter's syndrome

A condition in which there is primary testicular failure associated with a chromosomal abnormality. Chromosome studies show most subjects have XXY sex chromosome construction but may less commonly have chromatin-negative form (XY karyotype). Mosaicism has been reported. It is associated with an increased incidence of diabetes mellitus and cancer of the breast

Incidence: About 1 in 600 newborn males

Clinical features:
1 Tall stature, mildly impaired IQ
2 Eunuchoid and slightly feminized habitus
3 Poor beard growth
4 Gynaecomastia
5 Testicular atrophy with poor Leydig cell function
6 Infertile

Diagnosis:
1 Chromosome studies
2 Serum FSH elevated. Serum LH elevated or normal. Plasma testosterone normal or low
3 Urinary gonadotrophin elevated, urinary 17α-keto-steroids reduced

Management: If testosterone-deficient treat with androgens

Congenital abnormalities of uncertain origin

Possible causes include:
1 Infection: 'TORCH' (Toxoplasma, Other, Rubella, Cytomegalovirus, Herpesvirus)

2   Hormones: Progesterone, cortisone

3   Drugs: Thalidomide, aminopterine, progestagens, testosterone, quinine, warfarin

4   Physical agents: X-rays and irradiation

5   Maternal illnesses such as diabetes mellitus and hypothyroidism

6   Deficiencies: Hypoxia, vitamin deficiencies

Associated factors: Other pointers to an increased chance of malformation:

1   Previous history or a family history of congenital abnormality

2   Hydramnios or oligohydramnios

3   Diabetes mellitus

4   Intrauterine growth-retardation

Types of congenital abnormalities

These are discussed in detail in the appropriate chapter

1   Nervous system (see Chapter 12):
    a   Anencephaly
    b   Microcephaly
    c   Hydrocephaly
    d   Spina bifida

2   Musculoskeletal system (see Chapter 6):
    a   Congenital dislocation of the hip
    b   Talipes

3   Gastrointestinal system (see Chapter 13):
    a   Cleft lip and palate
    b   Oesophageal atresia
    c   Pyloric stenosis
    d   Intestinal obstruction
    e   Meckel's diverticulum
    f   Hirschsprung's disease

g   Imperforate or ectopic anus
h   Exomphalos
i   Umbilical hernia
j   Prune belly syndrome

4   Cardiovascular system (see Chapter 8):
    a   Ventricular septal defect
    b   Atrial septal defect
    c   Patent ductus arteriosus
    d   Pulmonary stenosis
    e   Coarctation of the aorta
    f   Aortic stenosis
    g   Tetralogy of Fallot
    h   Translocation of the great vessels
    i   Tricuspid stenosis
    j   Total anomalous pulmonary venous drainage

5   Respiratory system (see Chapter 7):
    a   Choanal atresia
    b   Diaphragmatic hernia
    c   Congenital laryngeal stridor
    d   Tracheo-oesophageal fistula

6   Genitourinary tract (covered below):
    a   Hypospadias and epispadias
    b   Cryptorchidism
    c   Intersex
    d   Renal agenesis
    e   Polycystic renal disease
    f   Congenital valves of the posterior urethra
    g   Ectopic ureter
    h   Ectopia vesicae

Congenital abnormalities of the genitourinary tract
(Figure 5.1)

1   Hypospadias: Incidence 1 in 160 births. The urethral
    orifice opens on the ventral surface of the glans penis.
    A common abnormality that requires no surgical

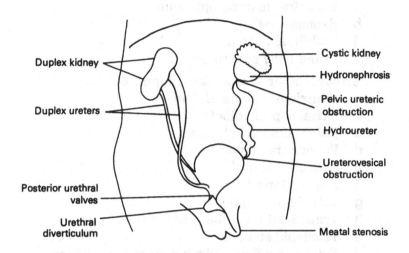

Figure 5.1 *Abnormalities of the urinary tract in infancy*

treatment unless there is some degree of 'anchoring' of the penis or meatal stenosis

2 Epispadias: Incidence 1 in 50 000 births. The urethral opening is on the dorsal (anterior) shaft of the penis.

3 Undescended testes (crytorchidism): The testes are in the scrotum in over 95% of full-term boys but this figure is less for pre-term boys. Undescended testes fall into two types:
   a Incomplete – testes stop somewhere along normal descent path
   b Ectopic testis – found in abnormal position

Complications of undescended testes:
   i Associated inguinal hernia
   ii Torsion of testis
   iii Malignant change in testis in later life
   iv Sterility – spermatogenesis is stimulated by lower temperature in scrotum

Treatment of undescended testes:

    i Testis may eventually descend – but not after 1 year of age

    ii If not descended by age 5 – orchidopexy

4 Pseudohermaphroditism: Many chromosomal aberrations can result in ambiguity of the external genitalia. In the female pseudohermaphrodite the genotype is XX, the gonads are ovaries but the external genitalia are virilized (masculinized). In the male pseudohermaphrodite the genotype is XY but the external genitalia are ambiguous or completely female. Testes can be present in abdomen or inguinal canal. Intersexuality is rare and true hermaphroditism is extremely rare

5 Renal agenesis: Absence of both kidneys is a rare and fatal condition. There is impaired fetal development and a characteristic frog-like appearance of the face (Potter's facies) with wide-set eyes, low-set ears and lung hypoplasia. The infants are usually male and are stillborn or die within hours of birth. Maternal oligohydramnios is sometimes present. Unilateral renal agenesis is compatible with a normal lifespan

6 Polycystic disease of the kidney: Infantile variety is usually bilateral and is inherited as an autosomal recessive characteristic. Abortive tubule formation renders kidney functionless. In 75% of cases, cystic changes are also found in bile ducts and liver

7 Congenital valves of the posterior urethra: Diagnosed by infrequent micturition or presence of a poor stream in the first week of life. Obstruction of the posterior urethra causes ureteral reflux, hydroureters and hydronephrosis. Treatment is surgical destruction of the valves through a urethroscope

8 Ectopic ureter: Usually arises from a duplex kidney and may open into vagina causing continual urinary incontinence

9   Ectopia vesicae: A very rare defect where the anterior wall of the bladder and abdominal wall are missing. The symphysis pubis is often absent and the pubic bones do not meet. The child is perpetually wet. Surgery is essential

Congenital abnormalities requiring prompt management

1   Diaphragmatic hernia:
Embryology: Failure of (usually) the left pleuroperitoneal canal to close. Results in abdominal viscera herniating into the thorax
Pathophysiology: Results in an early onset of respiratory distress
Clinical features:
    a   Respiratory distress soon after birth
    b   Abdomen may appear flat
Investigation: Presence of bowel shadows herniating into the thorax.
Management:
    a   Immediate intubation and artificial respiration followed by:
    b   Prompt surgical correction.

2   Oesophageal atresia:
See Figure 5.2

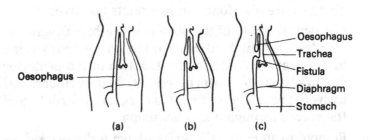

(a)   (b)   (c)

Figure 5.2   *Oesophageal atresia: (a) shows normal anatomy, (b) and (c) show two types of oesophageal atresia*

Antenatal diagnosis: Hydramnios may result from the fetus being unable to swallow amniotic fluid

Clinical features: The upper oesophageal pouch becomes filled with respiratory secretion. This results in aspiration of these fluids, and causes respiratory obstruction

Diagnosis: Passage of a radio-opaque catheter into the oesophagus will reveal the obstruction on X-ray

Management:
  a Aspiration of the upper oesophagus
  b Early surgical correction

3 Laryngeal atresia; laryngeal webs or stenosis:
  a Rare
  b Characterized by ineffectual inspiratory effort with or without stridor at birth
  c Managed by tracheostomy

4 Choanal atresia:
  a Pathology: Obstruction between nose and the pharynx. May be unilateral or bilateral
  b Features:
    i Breathing only possible through an open mouth
    ii Cyanosis and indrawing may occur while infant has its mouth closed, e.g. during feeding

5 Pierre-Robin syndrome:
  a In this syndrome there is hypoplasia of the mandible with cleft palate. The tongue may then roll backwards into the posterior pharynx and cause respiratory obstruction
  b Immediate management: Hold baby's face down and pull the tongue forward

6

Musculoskeletal System; Birth Injuries

CONGENITAL ABNORMALITIES OF THE MUSCULOSKELETAL SYSTEM

Congenital dislocation of the hip (CDH)

Anomaly of the hip joint where the head of the femur is partially or wholly displaced from the acetabulum

1 Aetiology:
  a Commoner in girls than boys; females: 1 in 600; males: 1 in 2500
  b Family history often present
  c Left hip more commonly affected than the right, although both may be affected
  d Positions in utero and after birth have been shown to be involved in the aetiology of CDH
  e Breech delivery
  f Reduced muscular tone, e.g. Down's syndrome

2 Diagnosis: Failure to diagnose the presence of a dislocated hip has serious orthopaedic consequences.

Diagnosis is by Barlow's modification of Ortolani's method – legs held at 45° of abduction with finger upon greater trochanter. If hip is dislocated a clunk is

79

heard or movement felt as the head of femur slides into the acetabulum. Three types of result are noted:

a   No movement of femoral head – normal hip
b   Femoral head moves forward – dislocated hip
c   Femoral head moves backwards – dislocatable hip

Confirm diagnosis by X-ray of hips

3   Management:
a   Under care of orthopaedic surgeon
b   A Von Rosen or Barlow splint is applied to keep the hips flexed and abducted for 3 months
c   Hip X-rays at 3 months

Talipes (Club foot)

1   Aetiology: Thought to be caused by posture of fetus *in utero*; genetic factors also play a part. May be bilateral.

2   Types:
a   Talipes equinovarus – commonest form of club foot with incurving of the whole foot and hyper-extension
b   Talipes calcanaeovalgus – flat or convex foot with a downward and inward-turning heel
c   Talipes metatarsovarus – forefoot angulates inwards

3   Management: Manipulation and strapping or a plaster cast

BIRTH INJURIES

Significant injury to the infant from a difficult or traumatic delivery is decreasing in incidence. Most traumatic deliveries can now be anticipated and avoided. Hypoxia is the commonest cause of 'cerebral' injury, but this is not usually regarded as an 'injury'.

Predisposing causes

1 Primiparity
2 Cephalopelvic disproportion
3 Post-term birth
4 Prematurity – compressibility of soft skull bones
5 Prolonged second stage of labour
6 Precipitate second stage of labour
7 Oligohydramnios

Head injuries

1 Moulding: A relative displacement of the bones of the skull vault occurring normally during delivery. It resolves in hours.

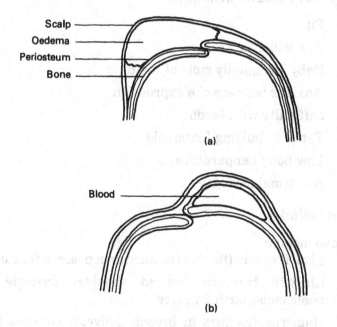

Figure 6.1   *(a) Caput succedaneum; (b) Cephalhaematoma*

2   Caput succedaneum: An oedematous swelling of soft tissues over the presenting portion of the scalp overlying the cervical os and lower uterine pole. It resolves in days (Figure 6.1a)

3   Cephalhaematoma: Haemorrhage beneath the periosteum. It resolves in weeks (Figure 6.1b)

4   Subaponeurotic haemorrhage: a coagulation defect is usually present and vitamin K should be given

5   Subdural haemorrhage: Haemorrhage from a bridging cerebral vein

6   Intracranial haemorrhage: Haemorrhage within brain tissue. Common cause of death or permanent neurological disability particularly in pre-term infants

Signs of cerebral irritation

1   Fits

2   Apnoeic attacks

3   Baby lies quietly most of the time

4   Anxious wide-awake expression

5   Difficulty with feeding

6   Tense or bulging fontanelle

7   Low body temperature

8   Abnormal crying

Bony injuries

These include

1   Skull fracture (fissure fracture or depressed fracture)

2   Clavicle fracture due to shoulder dystocia – commonest birth fracture

3   Humerus fracture in breech delivery: Observe for radial nerve paralysis

4 Femur fracture – very rare

5 Fracture of the spine: Observe for flaccid quadri-plegia – very rare.

Peripheral nerve injuries

1 Facial palsy (Bell's palsy):
   a Cause: pressure of forceps.blade on the facial nerve as the nerve emerges from the foramen ovale
   b Clinical features:
      i Lower motor neurone paralysis of the facial muscles
      ii Inability to close the eye on the affected side
   c Prognosis: Usually resolves by 2–3 months of age. Protection of the eye may be required

2 Brachial plexus palsy (Figure 6.2). Three clinical types occur:

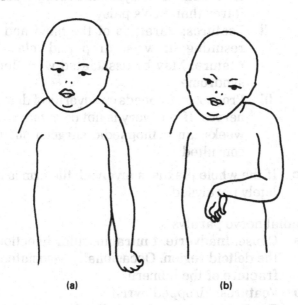

(a)   (b)

Figure 6.2 *(a) Erb's palsy; (b) Klumpke's palsy*

a Upper brachial plexus paralysis (Erb's palsy):
   i Cause: Uncommon condition caused by excessive traction on head during delivery. Compression of C5 and C6 fibres of the brachial plexus results
   ii Features: Limp arm with extended elbow, pronated forearm and flexed wrist – 'waiter's tip' posture
   iii Treatment: Splint with arm abducted, elbow flexed and wrist extended. With passive movements to maintain joint mobility
   iv Prognosis: Poor if no recovery within a month

b Lower brachial plexus paralysis (Klumpke's palsy):
   i Cause: Compression of C7 and C8 fibres during shoulder dystocia in breech delivery. Rarer than Erb's palsy
   ii Features: Paralysis of the hand and wrist resulting in wrist drop and 'claw-hand' posture. May be associated with Horner's syndrome
   iii Prognosis: Depends on severity of damage to nerves. If recovery is not complete within 6 weeks, an orthopaedic surgeon should be consulted

c If the whole plexus is involved, the arm is completely paralysed

3 Radial nerve paralysis:
a Cause: Inadvertent intramuscular injection into the deltoid region. Occasionally associated with fracture of the humerus
b Features: 'dropped' wrist
c Treatment: use cock-up splint for wrist drop

4 Sciatic nerve paralysis:
  a Cause: misplaced intramuscular injection in the buttock
  b Features: paralysis of the whole leg

7

Respiratory Problems

CONGENITAL ABNORMALITIES OF THE RESPIRATORY SYSTEM

1 Choanal atresia (see Chapter 5): Uncommon; obstruction of the nasal airway may produce respiratory difficulties

2 Diaphragmatic hernia (see Chapter 5): Occurs in about 1 in 2000 births. The stomach and other viscera usually herniate through the left diaphragm into the chest. Respiratory distress may result if the herniated volume is large.

3 Congenital laryngeal stridor: Extreme softness of the larynx ('floppy larynx') produces an inspiratory crowing noise

4 Tracheo-oesophageal fistula (see Chapter 5)

RESPIRATORY DISORDERS

Birth asphyxia

Lack of oxygen before, during or immediately after delivery is an important cause of stillbirth and neonatal death. The severity of birth asphyxia if present can be estimated by rating certain physical signs according to the Apgar scoring system, used in some centres. Assessment of the Apgar score should be determined 1 min after birth and 5 min after birth. A normal score should be 7 or above. A score of 4 or less indicates severe asphyxia and resuscitation measures should be employed immediately.

Apgar scoring

Sign	Score		
	0	*1*	*2*
Appearance	Blue or white	Blue limbs, pink body	All pink
Pulse	Absent	<100/min	>100/min
Grimace (reflex irritability)	None	Grimace	Cry
Activity	Flaccid	Some	Active
Respiration	Absent	Irregular	Good cry

Signs of respiratory distress in the newborn

1 Tachypnoea (>60/min)
2 Chest wall indrawing during inspiration and grunting or whining on expiration
3 Flaring of nostrils
4 Cyanosis
5 Use of accessory muscles of respiration

Causes of respiratory distress

1 Respiratory:
  a Respiratory distress syndrome (NB: This is the commonest cause of death in the first week of life)
  b Transient tachypnoea of the newborn
  c Meconium aspiration
  d Air leak – pneumothorax, pneumomediastinum
  e Pneumonia
  f Pulmonary haemorrhage

g Congenital abnormalities of the upper and lower airways, e.g. oesophageal atresia, diaphragmatic hernia

2 Cardiac:

   a Cardiac failure due either to congenital heart malformation or to an arrhythmia

Effects of hypoxia in the newborn

Physiological events	Clinical features	Treatment
Degree of respiratory effort →		
Hypoxia	'Blue asphyxia'	1 Clear the airway
Increased ventilation	1 Cyanosis	2 If blue and breathing: give facial oxygen
	2 Normal tone	3 If in primary apnoea, wait 2 min, and assess again. If pulse falling, then treat as case of terminal apnoea.
'Primary apnoea'	3 Normal pulse	
	4 Apnoea may be present	
Secondary	'White asphyxia'	1 If asphyxia severe and infant not breathing:
increased	1 Pallor, due to circulatory collapse	
ventilation	2 Falling tone	a Give assisted ventilation
'Last gasp'	3 Pulse falling, and below 100/min if untreated, leads to:	b Treat metabolic acidosis with slow infusion of $NaHCO_3$ or THAM intravenously through the umbilical vein
'Terminal apnoea'	a Mental defect	
Death	b Cerebral palsy	
	c Death	

Worsening degree of hypoxia (vertical, downward)

    b Cyanotic congenital heart disease
    c Cardiovascular depression by drugs

3 Anaemia:
    a Acute blood loss
    b Haemolytic disease of the newborn

4 Central nervous system:
    a Respiratory depression by drugs such as morphine or pethidine
    b Seizures and fits
    c Cerebral haemorrhage

5 Metabolic:
    a Hypoglycaemia
    b Methaemoglobinaemia – congenital or acquired

Causes of neonatal cyanosis

1 Peripheral cyanosis:
    a Traumatic or pressure cyanosis of head and neck in long deliveries
    b Poor peripheral circulation

2 Central cyanosis:
    a Respiratory causes:
        i   Primary or secondary apnoea
        ii Primary obstruction
        iii Respiratory distress syndrome
        iv Congenital lung or other intrathoracic abnormalities
        v Infection
    b Cardiovascular causes:
        i   Congenital heart disease
        ii Pulmonary hypertension
        iii Polycythaemia
        iv Methaemoglobinaemia

Signs of cyanosis

1 Dusky skin – blue-tinged lips, ears and fingertips
2 Blue tongue
3 Congestion of conjunctival and retinal blood vessels
4 Child sits in squatting position ⎫
5 Clubbing of fingers and toes ⎬ in later childhood

Causes of apnoea

1 Respiratory distress syndrome
2 Pulmonary haemorrhage
3 Other lung diseases
4 Upper airway obstruction
5 Systemic infection
6 Hypoglycaemia and hypercalcaemia
7 Cardiac failure
8 Intracranial haemorrhage
9 Iatrogenic – drugs

Investigation of apnoea

1 History and physical examination:
   a Maternal drugs
   b Maternal bleeding
   c Risk factors for infection (maternal fever, prolonged rupture of membranes, amnionitis)
   d Fetal asphyxia
   e Evidence of cardiorespiratory disease
   f Temperature
   g Association of apnoea with feeding
2 Laboratory investigation:
   a Haematocrit
   b Glucose, calcium, sodium

    c Arterial pH, P_{CO_2}, P_{O_2}
    d Blood culture, lumbar puncture, suprapubic bladder aspiration
    e Urine for metabolic screen (amino acids, organic acids)
    f Serum ammonia level
    g Magnesium

Treatment of apnoea

1 Treat underlying cause (e.g. sepsis, hyaline membrane disease, decreased glucose, decreased calcium, decreased blood pressure, PDA, seizure)

2 Temperature control:
    a Maintain environmental temperature
    b In a small infant, decrease heat loss

3 Avoid triggering reflexes:
    a Suction catheters
    b Tube-feed
    c Avoid cold stimulus to face

4 Maintain P_{O_2}

5 Maintain haematocrit

6 Frequent stimulation

7 Continuous positive airways pressure (CPAP)

8 Bag and mask ventilation

9 Mechanical ventilation

Causes of neonatal stridor

1 Laryngeal. Usually stridor is high-pitched:
    a Laryngeal web
    b Laryngeal stenosis
    c Laryngeal cyst or tumour
    d Vocal cord paralysis
    e Post-extubation laryngeal oedema

2   Tracheal. Stridor is low-pitched:
    a   Tracheal hypoplasia
    b   Tracheal compression by goitre, aberrant blood
        vessels or mediastinal tumours
3   Combined: Benign congenital laryngeal stridor
4   Metabolic: Hypocalcaemia

Note the following points:
1   Does the stridor occur in inspiration, expiration or
    both?
2   Is the stridor intermittent or constant?
3   Is cyanosis present?
4   Is the cry normal, hoarse or absent?

RESPIRATORY DISTRESS SYNDROME (HYALINE MEMBRANE DISEASE)

This is the single most common cause of death in the first
week of life (3.2 deaths/1000 live births). Respiratory
distress syndrome (RDS) is a fetal respiratory impairment
caused by a deficiency of surfactant, a substance normally
present lining the alveolar walls

Risk factors:
1   Prematurity
2   Birth by Caesarean section
3   Infants of diabetic mothers
4   Antepartum haemorrhage
5   Birth asphyxia
6   Commoner in males than in females
7   History of RDS in siblings
8   Rhesus disease

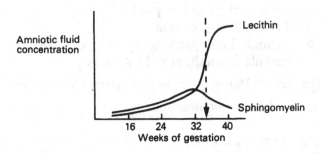

Figure 7.1   *Lecithin and sphingomyelin levels in amniotic fluid at different weeks of gestation*

Pathophysiology: Surfactant is a lipoprotein produced by Type II alveolar cells that reduces surface tension. Absence of surfactant causes alveolar collapse, transudation and fibrin deposition in the alveolar membranes. RDS occurs in pre-term infants, and is usually associated with an amniotic fluid lecithin/sphingomyelin (L/S) ratio of less than 2.0. (Figure 7.1):

L/S ratio	Clinical significance
1.5:1 or less	Immature lung
1.5:1 to 2:1	'Transitional' lung (repeat test in 1 week)
2:1 or greater	Mature lung

The ratio of 2:1 is normally attained by the 37th week of gestation. But some infants, particularly pre-term babies and those of diabetic mothers or born by Caesarean section, have mature L/S ratios but still get RDS; they are deficient in another surface-active protein. The L/S ratio can be ascertained in samples of amniotic fluid by amniocentesis

Clinical features: Infant usually premature with low Apgar scores at birth. Symptoms are usually obvious within ½–1 h of birth but in less severe cases, develop within first 4 h of postnatal life

1 Initially, respiration may be normal

2 Presence of two of the following triad developing before 4 h after birth:
   a Respiratory rate over 60/min
   b Subcostal or intercostal retraction ('see-saw' respiration)
   c Expiratory grunting, flaring of the alae nasi

3 Cardiovascular signs:
   a Tachycardia: 130 to 170/min
   b Central cyanosis
   c Oedema of hands and feet

4 Hypothermia – despite incubator care

Differential diagnosis:
   1 Meconium aspiration syndrome
   2 Transient tachypnoea of the newborn
   3 Pulmonary haemorrhage
   4 Congenital pneumonia
   5 Pneumothorax
   6 Congenital heart disease
   7 Persistent fetal circulation

Investigations:
   1 Radiology: 'Ground glass' lung fields and diffuse pulmonary collapse with air bronchograms stretching outside the cardiac shadow

   2 Biochemical: Fall in blood pH (may fall as low as 7.0) due to:
      a Respiratory acidosis because of CO_2 retention: arterial PCO_2 may rise to 10.5–13.5 kPa (80–100 mmHg))
      b Metabolic acidosis due to:
         i   Excessive respiratory effort
         ii Lactic acid accumulation

3 Hypoxia (arterial PO_2 may fall below 8 kPa (60 mmHg)) due to:
   a Poor ventilation
   b Right to left shunts

Prevention:
1 Adequate assessment of fetal gestational age during pregnancy and avoidance of premature delivery
2 Administration of glucocorticoids prior to birth for mothers with infants to be delivered before 32 weeks. Glucocorticoids accelerate lung maturity by inducing surfactant synthesis. Controlled studies of the benefit of corticosteroids on RDS are awaited. Beta-agonists have also been used

Treatment of respiratory distress syndrome:
1 General measures:
   a Place neonate in warm environment to reduce oxygen requirements, and correct hypothermia
   b Frequent monitoring of:
      i   Colour and respiration
      ii   Temperature: keep above 36 °C
      iii Pulse
      iv   Blood pressure: keep systolic arterial pressure above 40 mmHg
      v   Arterial pH, PO_2, PCO_2, HCO_3^- and base deficit: keep arterial PO_2 above 9 kPa (70 mmHg)
      vi   Blood glucose
      vii Blood electrolytes and calcium
      viii Blood bilirubin
      ix   Haematocrit
2 Correct hypoxia:
   a High ambient PO_2 to maintain umbilical artery PO_2 between 8 kPa and 12 kPa (60–90 mmHg)
   b PO_2 must be closely monitored, in view of the risk

of retrolental fibroplasia and subsequent blindness

c   If arterial PO_2 falls below 6.5 kPa (45 mmHg) or condition of neonate deteriorates, provide a continuous positive airways pressure (CPAP) of about 0.3–0.8 kPa (3–8 cm H_2O) to 'splint' alveoli open, especially during expiration

Complications of continuous positive airways pressure (CPAP):

   i   Pneumothorax
   ii   Intraventricular haemorrhage
   iii   Circulatory effects – reduced cardiac output due to decreased venous return
   iv   Disseminated intravascular coagulation (DIC)
   v   Intrapulmonary haemorrhage

3   Correct metabolic acidosis with 5% $NaHCO_3$ or Tris-hydroxyaminomethane (THAM) – this avoids sodium or CO_2 loading

4   Adequate nutrition. Oral feeding should be omitted for the first 2–3 days since many cases have a paralytic ileus

5   Antibiotics as required

Prognosis:

1   Most infants that do not suffer a major disturbance of their acid–base status for 3 days are likely to make a complete recovery with no further problems

2   Conversely, failure of the arterial PO_2 to respond to increasing inspired oxygen, or acidosis that is refractory to treatment, are poor prognostic indications

3   Less than 10% who were severely ill will develop neurological consequences or bronchopulmonary dysplasia (see page 101)

OTHER PULMONARY DISORDERS

Pulmonary haemorrhage

Causes:
1 Terminal event in respiratory distress syndrome
2 Fulminating infection
3 Disseminated intravascular coagulation
4 Severe hypothermia
5 Rhesus haemolytic disease
6 Congenital heart disease
7 Fluid overload
8 Oxygen toxicity

Clinical features:
1 Coughing of blood-stained secretions or aspiration of blood-stained material from the trachea
2 May only be a postmortem finding
3 X-ray usually shows homogeneously opaque lungs

Treatment: Symptomatic and supportive:
1 Give oxygen when required
2 Treat underlying cause if present
3 Transfuse blood
4 Ventilate – intermittent positive pressure ventilation (IPPV)
5 Control fluid balance
6 Sedation

Meconium aspiration syndrome

This results from the entry of meconium into the tracheo-bronchial tree. Bronchial obstruction may result, with secondary collapse of the lung

Pathophysiology (see Figure 7.2)

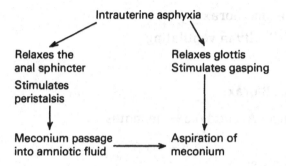

Figure 7.2 *Pathophysiology of meconium aspiration syndrome*

Clinical features:

1　Presence of meconium-stained amniotic fluid at birth

2　Baby often 'flat' at birth

3　Development of tachypnoea and cyanosis soon after birth

4　Obstruction may result in atelectasis of hyper-inflation

5　Coarse pulmonary infiltration on chest X-ray

6　Other conditions may coexist, e.g. pneumothorax and pneumonia

Management:
General management is the same as for respiratory distress syndrome

1　Deal with respiratory distress:
　　a　Laryngoscopy and endotracheal suction
　　b　Suction to remove inspired meconium with or without bronchial lavage

2　Prevent infection with antibiotic therapy

Complications:

1   Infection

2   Pneumothorax

3   Difficulty in ventilating

Pneumothorax

Incidence: Around 0.5% neonates

Risk factors:

1   Respiratory distress syndrome

2   Continuous positive airways pressure (CPAP)

3   Meconium aspiration syndrome

4   Coughing abnormalities

5   Tension cyst or lobar emphysema

6   Pulmonary interstitial emphysema

7   Congenital bullae

Clinical features:

1   Sudden deterioration in infant's condition – moderate or severe respiratory distress with increased PCO_2 and deteriorating PO_2

2   Signs of mediastinal shift may occur:
    a   Shift in apex
    b   Decreased air entry and percussion note on one side

Diagnosis:

1   Transillumination of each side of chest with a powerful light source

2   Chest X-ray – absence of normal lung markings

Management:

1 Insert an 'Intracath' needle with a three-way tap and large syringe to remove air

2 Underwater chest drainage

Intrauterine (congenital) pneumonia

Pathophysiology: Due to either blood-borne or ascending infection, usually by β-haemolytic streptococci

Risk factors:

1 Prolonged labour over 24 hours

2 Prolonged rupture of membranes

3 Maternal infection

Clinical features:

1 Features of birth asphyxia at delivery

2 Respiratory distress and/or apnoea

3 Hypothermia

Management:

1 Treat hypoxia

2 Chest X-ray

3 Blood culture

4 Deal with infective cause with appropriate antibiotic – intravenous penicillin and intramuscular gentamicin

Chronic lung disease of the neonate

Examples of chronic lung disease of the newborn include bronchopulmonary dysplasia and the Wilson–Mikity syndrome. This account is over-simplified.

Aetiology:

1 Assisted ventilation using a positive pressure machine

2 Respiratory distress syndrome

3 Extreme prematurity

Diagnosis:

1 Bronchopulmonary dysplasia usually starts earlier in infants than the Wilson–Mikity syndrome

2 Both conditions are characterized by tachypnoea, dyspnoea and oxygen dependency

3 Both conditions are characterized by cystic changes on chest X-ray – the so-called 'bubbly lung'

Treatment:

1 Supportive management with oxygen

2 Consider respiratory support, e.g. continuous positive airways pressure (CPAP)

3 Chest physiotherapy when indicated

4 Digoxin and diuretics for cor pulmonale when indicated

5 Corticosteroids may be used for severe cases

6 Long-term prognosis good if infants survive first few months of life

Retrolental fibroplasia

Premature infants receiving an oxygen concentration above 30% are at risk of retrolental fibroplasia. Documented cases exist where there is no history of increased inspired oxygen

Prevention:

1 The oxygen concentration should be closely monitored and all premature infants that have been

treated with oxygen should have an ophthalmological examination prior to discharge

2 Vitamin E administration

Detection: Indirect ophthalmoscopy through a maximally dilated pupil

Pathophysiology: This is a retinopathy that may:
1 Remain stationary

2 Regress

3 Proceed to progressive cicatricial disease with eventual retinal detachment. In advanced cases blindness results from the formation of a dense retrolental white mass.

8

Cardiovascular Problems

CLINICAL SIGNS OF CARDIAC DISEASE

1 Respiratory distress and cyanosis
 For further details see Chapter 7

2 Cardiac murmur
 a Most cardiac murmurs heard in the first day of life are benign
 b Conversely, absence of a murmur does not exclude cardiac disease
 c Loud murmurs are more likely to be significant, but small defects can cause a loud murmur
 d In the absence of other cardiovascular signs, a murmur can be investigated by chest X-ray, ECG and full blood count
 e If heart sounds are loudest on the right side, the likeliest causes are:
  i True dextrocardia
  ii Pneumothorax
  iii Diaphragmatic hernia

3 Bradycardia. This may result from:
 a Prolonged apnoea
 b Congenital heart block
 c Severe hypocalcaemia

4 Tachycardia. This may result from:
  a Crying
  b Pyrexia
  c Incipient cardiac failure
  d Atrial tachycardia (over 200 beats/min)

5 Cardiac failure: Clinical features are:
  a Tachycardia and tachypnoea especially on feeding
  b Liver enlargement
  c Oedema
  d Lung crepitations
  e Cardiomegaly on chest X-ray
  f Sweating

6 Enlarged heart on chest X-ray. This may result from:
  a Congestive cardiac failure
  b Pericardial effusion
  c Congenital myocarditis
  d Endocardial fibroelastosis
  e Glycogen storage disease

7 Oedema:
  a Generalized oedema may result from:
    i Cardiac failure
    ii Renal disease
    iii Cold injury
    iv Hypoproteinaemia
    v Fluid overload
    vi Prematurity
    vii *In utero* closure of foramen ovale
    viii Hydrops fetalis
  b Local causes of oedema (listed here for completeness) are:
    i Birth trauma
    ii Oedema of the extremities in Turner's syndrome
    iii Thrombosis of inferior vena cava
    iv Milroy's disease

CONGENITAL CARDIAC DISEASE

Classification

1   Abnormalities of the atrial septum: Ostium secundum defect. A large opening between the left and right atrium. It results from either excessive absorption of the embryonic septum primum or inadequate development of the septum secundum. It may result in considerable intracardiac shunting of blood

2   Abnormalities of the atrioventricular canal:
   a   Persistent atrioventricular canal: A failure of the endocardial cushions to close results in a persistent atrioventricular channel. There is a defect in the cardiac septum in both the atria and the ventricles
   b   Ostium primum defect: This results from incomplete fusion of the endocardial cushions. It results in a defect in the atrial septum but the interventricular septum is intact. Usually there are also defects in both mitral and tricuspid valves
   c   Tricuspid atresia: This results from obliteration of the right atrioventricular orifice. There is a fusion of the tricuspid valves. Associated abnormalities usually include atrial septal defect, ventricular septal defect, underdeveloped right ventricle and a hypertrophied left ventricle

3   Abnormalities of the interventricular septum: Defects of the membraneous septum result in ventricular septal defect

4   Abnormalities of the truncus and conus:
   a   Tetralogy of Fallot: Caused by an anterior displacement of the truncoconal septum resulting in an unequal division of the conus. This results in:

      i   A narrow right ventricular outflow region
     ii A defect in the interventricular septum
    iii An 'over-riding' aorta arising from both ventricular cavities
     iv Hypertrophy of the right ventricle

b Persistent truncus arteriosus: A failure of the spiral ridges to descend and fuse results in the pulmonary artery arising some distance above the origin of the undivided truncus. This condition is associated with ventricular septal defects.

c Transposition of the great vessels: The truncoconal septum descends straight downward instead of taking a spiral course. As a result, the aorta originates from the right ventricle and the pulmonary artery from the left ventricle. In addition there may be an associated ventricular septal defect and patent ductus arteriosus. The latter is the access route to the lungs

5 Abnormalities of the semilunar valves:
   a Valvular stenosis of the pulmonary artery
   b Aortic valvular stenosis

6 Congenital anomalies of the great arteries:
   a Patent ductus arteriosus
   b Coarctation of the aorta
   c Double aortic arch

Pathophysiology

Congenital cardiac disease can be divided into three groups:

1 Left-to-right shunts present: Acyanotic group
   a Cyanosis is usually absent
   b There often is a harsh systolic murmur
   c Increased pulmonary markings on chest X-rays. Examples:

    i Ventricular septal defect
    ii Atrial septal defect
    iii Patent ductus arteriosus
    Left-to-right shunts may change to right-to-left shunts if resistance rises on the right side:

2 Right-to-left shunt: Cyanotic group. Cyanosis is present. Examples include:
    a Tetralogy of Fallot
    b Transposition of the great vessels
    c Tricuspid atresia
    d Persistent truncus arteriosus

3 'Blocked pipes' (No shunt present): These result in cardiovascular disability owing to abnormally high pressures produced in certain chambers. Examples:
    a Aortic stenosis
    b Pulmonary stenosis
    c Coarctation of the aorta

Investigation of congenital cardiac disease

1 General principles are:
    a Murmurs in the first 24 h are often benign and should be reassessed later, in the meantime, monitor pulse, respiration and weight gain
    b Differentiation from pulmonary disease can be made by the hyperoxia test: in this test, exposure of the baby to 100% oxygen causes no clinical improvement in cyanotic congenital heart disease nor improvement in blood gases
    c Definitive diagnosis usually requires a cardiological opinion

2 Basic investigations are:
    a Chest X-ray
    b Electrocardiogram
    c Blood pressure measurements
    d Haematocrit from heel-prick sample

3 Cardiac catheterization and angiography
Uses:
  a Produce an accurate anatomical diagnosis
  b Determination of the size of flows and shunts and
other cardiac parameters
  c Determination of oxygen saturation in different
chambers

Management of congenital cardiac disease

1 Investigation and assessment. This will require a
cardiological opinion:
  a Chest X-ray
  b Cardiac catheterization with angiographic
studies

2 Management of cardiac failure:
  a Risk groups:
    i Coarctation of the aorta
    ii Transposition of the great vessels
    iii Patent ductus arteriosus
    iv Aortic atresia
    v Supraventricular tachycardia
    vi Ventricular septal defect
  NB: other causes of cardiac failure include:
    i Myocarditis
    ii Endocardial fibroelastosis
    iii Profound anaemia, e.g. in hydrops fetalis
(see Chapter 9)
  b Medical treatment:
    i Supportive management:
     • Warm and humidified oxygen should
be given to relieve cyanosis
     • Tube-feeding: if severe oedema is
present give a low sodium milk
     • Nurse infant in sitting-up or semi-
prone position

- Control sodium intake
- Correct all associated metabolic problems

ii Digitalization: Careful attention needed to ascertain dose of digoxin. The digitalizing dose is around 50 μg/kg body weight, intravenously or intramuscularly over the first 24 h. The maintenance dose is around 20–25% of the digitalizing dose. Heart rate and ECG changes should be monitored and the drug stopped temporarily if the pulse rate falls below 100/min

iii Diuresis:
- Initially: frusemide, approximately 0.5 mg/kg to promote diuresis
- Maintenance diuretic: e.g. bendrofluazide 2.5 mg every 1–2 days
  Usually K$^+$ supplementation may be needed

3 Assessment for surgical treatment

NOTES ON SPECIFIC TYPES OF CONGENITAL HEART DISEASE (CHD)

NB: Some of the discussion may refer to childhood, that is, after the neonatal period
1 Ventricular septal defect (VSD) (Figure 8.1)
Pathophysiology: Defect in ventricular septum that results in communication between ventricles. Failure of the embryonic interventricular foramen to close. At least 20–25% of all congenital heart disease, and may be associated with trisomies 13, 18 and 21.
Clinical features:
a Small defect: Asymptomatic. Murmur may be loud and harsh or may be only grade II in intensity
b Moderate defect: Congestive heart failure,

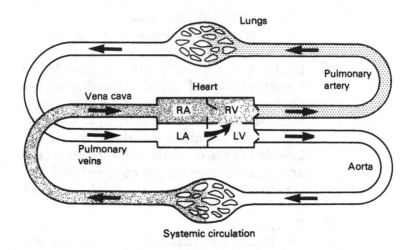

Figure 8.1   *Ventricular septal defect (VSD)*

pneumonia, growth failure, loud pansystolic murmur heard best at lower left sternal border

c   Large defect: Same as with moderate defect except that congestive heart failure and pneumonia are more likely to occur. Also an apical mitral flow murmur.

Investigation:

a   Chest film may be normal or show enlarged heart with increased pulmonary vasculature

b   Electrocardiogram may be normal or show left ventricular, right ventricular, or combined hypertrophy

c   Cardiac catheterization

Complications:

a   Pulmonary vascular obstructive disease: In cases of long-standing shunt; eventually shunt reversal with right-to-left shunt cyanosis

b   Congestive heart failure: During early months of life pulmonary vascular resistance decreases resulting in increased left-to-right shunting with overload of left heart and left ventricular failure.

Cardiac failure, when it occurs, usually does so at 1–6 months of age

c Bacterial endocarditis:

Management:

a As many as 50% of small and moderate defects may close spontaneously – usually first 2 years of life

b Initially treat medically (see patent ductus arteriosus)

c If there is evidence of increasing pulmonary vascular resistance, early surgery is required.

d Elective repair at 2–5 years; but surgery not indicated for small defects.

2 Atrial septal defect (ASD) (Figure 8.2)

Pathophysiology: Defect in atrial septum – either in middle or upper part. Accounts for around 12% of cases of CHD

Clinical features: Findings usually only on clinical examination where there may be:

a Ejection systolic murmur

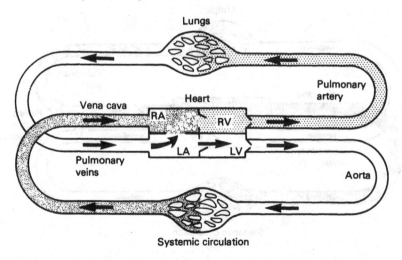

Figure 8.2 *Atrial septal defect (ASD)*

b If shunting is large, there may additionally be a mid-diastolic murmur at the left sternal edge and a fixed splitting of the second sound

Investigation:

a ECG may show right ventricular hypertrophy and right bundle branch block

b Chest X-ray shows enlarged right atrium and ventricle and enhanced pulmonary markings

c Catheterization may show increased right atrial PO_2

Surgical closure: Indicated only if pulmonary blood flow greatly exceeds systemic blood flow. Normally asymptomatic in childhood

3 Patent ductus arteriosus (PDA) (Figure 8.3)
Pathophysiology:

a Persistence of the sixth aortic arch, which maintains its distal connection with the dorsal aorta. Normally closes functionally on first day and anatomically in first year

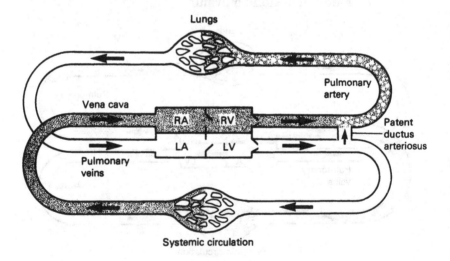

Figure 8.3   *Patent ductus arteriosus (PDA)*

b Usually shunt is from aorta to pulmonary artery resulting in increased flow to lungs and volume overload of left side of heart

Clinical features: Depend on age of patient and size of shunt. Classic murmur is continuous ('machinery murmur'), maximal at left sternal border in second, third intercostal spaces. During first 6 months of life, diastolic component may be absent

  a Small patent ductus: Asymptomatic murmur

  b Moderate patent ductus:

    i Poor feeding, irritability, tachypnoea, slight retardation of growth, bounding peripheral pulses

    ii Electrocardiogram may show left ventricular hypertrophy. Increased pulmonary vascularity on X-ray

  c Large patent ductus:

    i Always symptomatic. Same as with moderate patent ductus plus recurrent pneumonia, rales on auscultation, heart failure

    ii With congestive heart failure, murmur may become fainter

    iii Electrocardiogram typically shows left ventricular hypertrophy

    iv Chest film shows cardiomegaly with hypervascularity of lung fields

Investigations:

  a Electrocardiogram, X-ray, echocardiogram

  b Cardiac catheterization

Complications:

  a Congestive heart failure

  b Pulmonary vascular disease with pulmonary hypertension

  c Subacute bacterial endocarditis

  d Aneurysm of ductus

  e Growth failure

  f Recurrent pneumonia

Management:
a   Restrict fluids
b   Keep haematocrit above 45% (to prevent heart failure)
c   Diuretics
d   Indomethacin: Inhibits prostaglandin synthesis; permanent closure more likely if therapy started in first 10 days of life; full response in very immature infants less likely; monitor urine output. Contraindications: Bleeding, reduced renal function, disorders of bilirubin metabolism.
e   Surgery if medical management fails.

4   Pulmonary stenosis:
Pathophysiology: Obstruction to outflow from the right ventricle. In most cases this is due to a valvular lesion; occasionally the obstruction is subvalvular (infundibular)
Accounts for under 10% of cases of CHD
Clinical features:
a   May be asymptomatic in mild cases. If severe, heart failure may result. Cyanosis indicates associated right-to-left shunt through the foramen ovale
b   Loud ejection murmur at left base, radiating to the back. Soft second sound
Investigation:
a   ECG may be normal. In severe cases there may be right ventricular hypertrophy and/or right axis deviation
b   Chest X-ray may reveal right-sided enlargement in severe cases. There may also be post-stenotic dilatation of the pulmonary artery
c   Catheterization shows increased right ventricular pressure and normal or reduced pressures in the pulmonary artery. Elevation of right ventricular pressure usually correlates with amount of hypertrophy

d Angiocardiography may be required to localize the site of obstruction

Management: Surgical correction is indicated if the peak pressure drop across the stenosis exceeds around 70 torr

5 Coarctation of the aorta:
Pathophysiology: Narrowing of the aorta may occur either beyond the ductus arteriosus, or proximally, in the aortic arch. Commoner in males but accounts for less than 5–10% of all cases of CHD. Common in Turner's syndrome
Clinical features:
   a May be asymptomatic or result in congestive heart failure in infancy, and hypertension in later life
   b Examination may reveal systolic murmur over back and delayed or absent femoral pulses
   c Increased blood pressure as measured in arms
Investigation:
   a ECG shows right bundle branch block
   b Chest X-ray: normal pulmonary markings and normal heart size. Cardiac enlargement and rib-notching are later signs
Management: Surgical correction if narrowing is significant, i.e. if hypertension develops, in later life

6 Aortic stenosis
Pathophysiology: Obstructed left ventricular outflow usually due to valvular narrowing. Accounts for about 5% of cases of CHD
Clinical features:
   a Asymptomatic if mild. May cause dyspnoea if severe
   b Loud systolic ejection murmur at right base, radiating to neck
Investigation:
   a ECG: left ventricular hypertrophy

b Chest X-ray may be normal – even in severe cases

c Catheterization: elevated right ventricular pressure

d Check calcium status

Management: Surgery indicated only for moderate to severe cases, significant symptoms, or if transaortic pressure gradient is over 50 torr

7 Tetralogy of Fallot (Figure 8.4)

Pathophysiology:

a Ventricular septal defect

b Pulmonary stenosis, often infundibular rather than valvular

c Overriding aorta

d Right ventricular hypertrophy

Accounts for around 10% of cases of CHD and up to 60% of cases of cyanotic heart disease

Clinical features:

a Symptoms of cyanosis, dyspnoea and 'squatting'

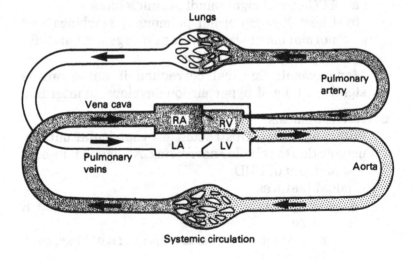

Figure 8.4   *Tetralogy of Fallot*

spells usually occur after 2–3 months of age. Heart failure is rare in childhood

b On examination, loud systolic murmur along left sternal edge and soft second sound. Cyanosis may be present

Investigation:

a ECG may show right axis deviation and right ventricular hypertrophy

b Chest X-ray shows attenuated pulmonary markings, small heart and diminished pulmonary conus

c Catheterization shows diminished pulmonary artery pressure, and equal pressures in right and left ventricles. Right-to-left shunt may compromise PO_2 in aorta. Angiocardiography is needed to demonstrate anatomy

Management:

a In infants: palliative aortic-pulmonary shunt with definitive surgical correction in childhood

b Presentation in early childhood: full surgical correction

8 Transposition of the great arteries (Figure 8.5)
Pathophysiology:

a Aorta arising from right ventricle

b Pulmonary artery arising from the left ventricle

c Communication between right and left side – atrial septal defect, ventricular septal defect, or patent ductus arteriosus, must exist to allow survival

Accounts for up to 5% of cases of CHD

Clinical features:

a Presentation in the neonatal period with progressive cyanosis, tachypnoea and congestive cardiac failure

b On examination, cyanosis, dyspnoea. Murmurs may be absent

Investigation:

a Right axis deviation and moderate right ventricular hypertrophy on ECG

b Chest X-ray shows increased pulmonary perfusion, cardiomegaly – 'egg-shaped' heart

c Catheterization – high pressures (systemic levels) in right ventricle. Low PO_2 levels. Angiocardiography needed to demonstrate anatomy of abnormalities

Management:

a Investigation and management should be undertaken promptly as symptoms may progress rapidly. Balloon-catheter atrial septostomy (Rashkind operation) or operative production of atrial septal defect may be needed as life-saving procedure. Early full correction carries a high mortality

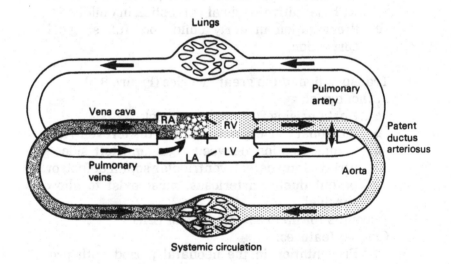

Figure 8.5 *Transposition of the great vessels, showing the possible associated shunts: atrial septal defect, ventricular septal defect and patent ductus arteriosus*

b This can be followed by complete correction using intra-atrial venous transposition

9 Tricuspid atresia:
Pathophysiology: Stenotic or absent tricuspid valve. Where absent there is an associated ventricular septal defect with a right-to-left shunt. Accounts for less than 2% of cases of CHD
Clinical features:
  a Early development of cyanosis and tachypnoea in infancy
  b On examination systolic murmur due to associated septal defect may occur
  c Giant jugular 'a' waves
  d Enlarged liver
Investigation:
  a ECG shows left axis deviation and left ventricular hypertrophy
  b Chest X-ray shows decreased pulmonary vascular markings and small size of heart. May be confused with tetralogy of Fallot
  c Catheterization. Catheter will pass from right atrium to left side of heart and decreased PO_2 levels are found.
  d Angiocardiography needed to demonstrate abnormality
Management: Right ventricle usually hypoplastic, which makes correction not feasible. Palliation by aortic–pulmonary or subclavian–pulmonary shunt

10 Total anomalous pulmonary venous return
Pathophysiology:
  a All pulmonary veins enter the right atrium
  b Associated atrial septal defect
Accounts for about 1% of CHD
Clinical features:
  a Congestive heart failure may develop early in infancy. Mild to moderate cyanosis

    b Soft systolic murmur, with diastolic murmur at left sternal border

    c Third and fourth sounds

Investigation:

    a ECG: right axis deviation and right ventricular hypertrophy

    b Chest X-ray – increased pulmonary vascular markings. Enlarged right atria and ventricle

    c Catheterization – normal right ventricle and pulmonary arterial pressures; complete mixing of venous and arterial blood, hence PO_2 will be equal in atria, pulmonary artery and aorta

Management: Complete correction in most cases

DISTURBANCES OF CARDIAC RHYTHM

Causes of bradycardia

1 Sinus bradycardia

    Features:

    a Rare

    b Normal PQRST complexes; heart rate below 100/min

    Associations:

    a Congenital cardiac disease

    b Raised intracranial pressure

    c Hypertension

    d Hyperkalaemia

    Management: Treat underlying cause, if present

2 Congenital heart block

    Rare: may be congenital or secondary to or associated with myocarditis, rheumatic fever, digoxin therapy, etc. Cases have been reported following maternal systemic lupus erythematosus during pregnancy

    Management:

    a Heart rate above 50/min – may be asymptomatic and only need to be monitored for heart rate and respiratory rate

b Heart rate below 50/min – may require chrono-tropic agent to deal with respiratory distress and heart failure. Persistent bradycardia may require pacemaker implantation

3 First-degree atrioventricular heart block
Features:
   a Prolonged PR interval; P and QRS complex normal; normal heart rate
   b May be associated with a conducting system disorder, or with digoxin treatment
Management: No specific treatment

4 Second-degree atrioventricular heart block
Types:
   a Mobitz type I (Wenckebach block): Cycles of progressive lengthening of PR interval followed by a failure of appearance of the QRS complex
   b Mobitz type II: Constant PR interval, but with intermittent failure (2:1, 3:1 etc) for the beat to conduct to the ventricles
      These may reflect a congenital conducting disorder, or digoxin treatment
Management: Treat underlying condition, if any. If severe cardiovascular consequences, treat with isoprenaline to increase the heart rate

5 Third-degree atrioventricular block
Features: Dissociation of the atrial (P) wave and the ventricular (QRS) electrical and mechanical activity. The effective ventricular rate may then vary between 50 and 100 beats/min
Associations:
   a Digoxin toxicity
   b Congenital heart disease
   c Congenital conduction disturbance
Management:
   a If the ventricular rate is over 50/min and the neonate is asymptomatic – no specific treatment

b If the rate is below 50/min and/or the neonate is symptomatic with respiratory distress or cardiac failure, treat with isoprenaline and implant pacemaker if block is persistent

Causes of tachycardia

1 Sinus tachycardia:
   Features: Common; heart rate 140 to 200/min. Normal PQRS
   Associations: Response to stress, pyrexia, hypovolaemia
   Management: Treat the cause

2 Paroxysmal atrial tachycardia:
   Features:
     a Common; heart rate 200–300/min. Few if any P waves
     b May be first detected *in utero*
   Associations:
     a Wolf–Parkinson–White syndrome
     b Structural congenital heart disease
   Management:
     a Detected *in utero*: may result in fetal congestive heart failure or hydrops fetalis. Treat mother with digoxin and plan as early a delivery as is permitted by lecithin and sphingomyelin levels in amniotic fluid
     b In the infant:
       i Vagal stimulation – e.g. pressing on fontanelle
       ii Digitalization
       iii Cardioversion if condition deteriorates

3 Atrial flutter:
   Features:
     a Uncommon – flutter waves are coarse with a regular sawtooth appearance

b Fairly well tolerated but often associated with congenital heart disease

Management:

a Digitalization to increase degree of AV block

b Restoration to sinus rhythm using propranolol; cardioversion if cardiovascular function deteriorates

4 Atrial fibrillation:

Features:

a Fibrillation on ECG; irregular ventricular response at 120–250 beats/min

b May be associated with congenital heart disease, e.g. atrial septal defect and patients with large atria

Management:

a Slow ventricular rate by digitalization

b Cardioversion if necessary

5 Supraventricular tachycardia:

Features: Normal QRS, but no preceding P wave; heart rate 130–140/min

Associations:

a Digoxin toxicity

b Electrolyte or hypoxic disturbance

Management:

a Treat the underlying cause

b Vagal stimulation

6 Ventricular tachycardia:

Features:

a Rare; rate at 120–240/min

b P waves absent. QRS broad and misshapen

c Requires prompt treatment – greatly compromises cardiac function

Association:

a Cardiac failure

b Gross electrolyte or hypoxic disturbance

c Digoxin overdose

Management:
> **a** Lignocaine loading infusion to treat acutely. Consider oral antiarrythmic therapy (e.g. procainamide; disopyramide, propranolol) if ventricular tachycardia recurs after withdrawal of lignocaine
> **b** Cardioversion, if necessary

7 Ventricular fibrillation:
Features: Dying infant, coarse irregular ECG activity. No effective cardiac function
Management:
> **a** Cardiac massage
> **b** Lignocaine, 1 mg/kg, infusion
> **c** Cardioversion
> **d** Manage underlying cause

Ectopic beats

1 Atrial ectopic beats; junctional ectopic beats:
Features: Common, but usually benign. Abnormal or absent P waves, short PR interval and normal QRS
Associations: May occur in normal infant, or in association with digoxin toxicity, or hypoxia
Management: Treat the underlying cause

2 Ventricular ectopic beats:
Features: Uncommon. Abnormal QRS complex with no preceding P wave
Associations:
> **a** Digoxin toxicity
> **b** Hypoxic or electrolyte disturbance

Management:
> **a** Treat the underlying cause
> **b** If more than 10/min treat with lignocaine infusion

9

Neonatal Jaundice; Haematological Problems

NEONATAL JAUNDICE

About 50% of neonates show clinical jaundice. This is associated with increased blood levels of unconjugated bilirubin (but see below) and produces the characteristic golden-yellow clinical appearance of the baby's skin. Jaundice is not detectable until serum bilirubin levels rise

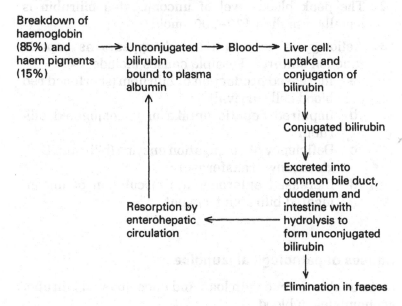

Breakdown of haemoglobin (85%) and haem pigments (15%) ——> Unconjugated bilirubin bound to plasma albumin ——> Blood ——> Liver cell: uptake and conjugation of bilirubin

Conjugated bilirubin

Excreted into common bile duct, duodenum and intestine with hydrolysis to form unconjugated bilirubin

Resorption by enterohepatic circulation <———

Elimination in faeces

Figure 9.1   *Summary of bilirubin metabolism and excretion*

above 75 μmol/l. Bilirubin conjugation is of clinical importance as lipid-soluble unconjugated bile salts are neurotoxic, and can cause kernicterus

NB: **a**   Mild jaundice – serum bilirubin 75–175 μmol/l

     b   Moderate jaundice – serum bilirubin 175–250 μmol/l

     c   Severe jaundice – serum bilirubin above 250 μmol/l

'Physiological jaundice' in the newborn

1   Appears in an otherwise healthy baby between the 3rd and 7th days of life. The liver and spleen are not enlarged

2   The peak blood level of unconjugated bilirubin is usually less than 170–200 μmol/l

3   Aetiology is uncertain but disappears as hepatic function matures. Possible causes include:

    a   Increased production of bilirubin (shortened red blood cell survival)

    b   Impaired hepatic uptake of unconjugated bilirubin

    c   Deficiency of conjugation enzyme (bilirubin UDP glucuronyl transferase)

    d   Increased enterohepatic circulation of unconjugated bilirubin from gut

Causes of pathological jaundice

Liver unable to cope with load and unconjugated bilirubin accumulates in blood

1   Overproduction of bilirubin:

    a   Haemolytic disease:

       i   Rhesus or ABO haemolytic disease

    ii Hereditary spherocytosis
    iii Erythrocyte enzyme defects and haemo-
        globin defects
  b Polycythaemia:
    i Small-for-dates
    ii Down's syndrome
    iii Materno-fetal transfusion
    iv Infants of diabetic mothers
  c Haemorrhage:
    i Bruising
    ii Internal haemorrhage
  d Increased enterohepatic re-circulation
    i Poor fluid intake – increasing intestinal
        transmit time and allowing greater bilirubin
        absorption
    ii Paralytic ileus
  e Competition for binding sites on plasma proteins

2 Decreased bilirubin secretion:
  a Breast milk jaundice
  b Congenital hypothyroidism
  c Inborn errors of metabolism; e.g. galactosaemia
  d Obstructive jaundice; e.g. congenital biliary
    atresia, cystic fibrosis
  e Crigler–Najjar syndrome
  f Some drugs

3 Combined bilirubin overproduction and under-
secretion:
  a Pre-term baby
  b Neonatal sepsis
  c Neonatal hepatitis
  d Roter and Dubin–Johnson syndromes

4 Bile duct atresia: Usually present after 2nd week.
Produces an obstructive jaundice with a poor
prognosis

General features of pathological jaundice

Any one of the following:
1 An unwell baby
2 Jaundice appearing within the first 24 h after birth
3 Jaundice persisting after the 10th day after birth
4 Jaundice recurring after a partial recovery
5 Total bilirubin level greater than 250 μmol/l (approximately 15 mg%)

Investigation of neonatal jaundice

1 Suspected haemolytic jaundice:
   a Haemoglobin level and haematocrit
   b Blood grouping of both mother and baby
   c Direct Coombs test
   d Blood film: in particular reticulocyte count
   e Special studies as indicated, e.g.:
      i Haemoglobin electrophoresis. However, note that diseases such as thalassaemia do not present until about 3 months when HbF synthesis is being superseded
      ii Osmotic fragility of red cells
      iii Titre of anti-A or anti-B haemolysins in maternal or baby blood
      iv Glucose-6-phosphate dehydrogenase estimation
2 Non-haemolytic jaundice:
   a Total white cell count and differential count; platelet count
   b Serology: IgM levels
   c Bacteriological tests: of urine, blood, skin and cerebrospinal fluid
   d Special tests as indicated:
      i Viral cultures
      ii Liver function tests

   iii Thyroid function tests
   iv Serum α_1-antitrypsin
   v Sweat sodium concentration, but unreliable
     test in newborn
   vi Urine, for reducing substances to exclude
     galactosaemia

Complications of neonatal jaundice

1 Bilirubin encephalopathy: This reflects brain cell
death due to elevated levels of bilirubin in extracellular fluid. Levels of bilirubin above 340 μmol/l
cause brain cell death
Clinical features:
   a Severely jaundiced; level of bilirubin depends on
     size of infant and acid–base balance
   b Lethargy
   c Disinclination to feed
   d 'Sunsetting' appearance of eyes
   e Convulsions, opisthotonus
   f Eventually: coma
Prognosis: Recovery is possible but frequently there
are residual neurological signs, viz. high-tone nerve
deafness and athetoid cerebral palsy

2 Kernicterus: Deposition of bilirubin in the brain
especially in the basal ganglia and hippocampus.
Kernicterus appears after a period of jaundice which
may be only a few hours
Clinical features:
   a Permanent brain damage following bilirubin
     encephalopathy may result in:
     i Mental retardation
     ii Nerve deafness
     iii Athetoid cerebral palsy
   b Green staining of dentition

c 'Sunsetting' appearance of eyes
Prognosis: Treatment of kernicterus is not possible
Treatment of neonatal jaundice is discussed on page
138

RHESUS HAEMOLYTIC DISEASE

The 'Rhesus factor' (Rh) is a complex antigen residing on
the membrane of erythrocytes of 'Rhesus-positive'
persons. It was first described in 1940. Incompatibility
may occur if a Rh-negative mother carries a fetus with Rh-
positive antibodies on its erythrocytes. At delivery, Rh-
positive fetal erythrocytes may enter the maternal circulation and stimulate production of anti-Rh antibodies.
These are principally IgG immunoglobulins and can therefore be transported across the placenta (from mother to
fetus) in a subsequent or even the same pregnancy to
combine with Rh antigens on the fetal erythrocytes,
causing red cell haemolysis. This triggers a series of patho-
logical events that may result in injury to, or the death of
the fetus.

Pathophysiology

Genetics: There are six Rh antigens (C, D, E, c, d, e) of which
the D and d are the most important immunologically. Rh-C,
D and E are dominant and Rh-c, d and e are genetic recessives. The 'D' antigen is present in 85% of Caucasians,
95% of Blacks and 99% of Orientals. In the UK population
15% of females are Rh-negative, i.e. they have two recessive genes (i.e. d–d)

Rhesus iso-immunization: If the mother is Rh-positive (her
genetic status would then be D–d or D–D), there is no risk
of immunization.

   If the mother is Rh-negative (d–d), and the father is Rh-
positive (D–d, D–D), he may give his wife a Rh-positive

child, and this may result in inoculation of the mother with Rh-positive antigen. The inoculation of Rh-positive antigen into the mother may arise from:

1 Transfusions with Rh-positive blood
2 Transplacental entry of Rh-positive antigen from a previous pregnancy or a previous abortion
3 Entry of Rh-positive antigen during the current pregnancy

It is rare for a first pregnancy to sensitize a woman. Before the introduction of prophylaxis, one in ten Rh-negative women became autoimmunized as a result of two such pregnancies.

Detection

1 History: In all pregnancies, enquire for:
    a History of previous Rh-haemolytic disease
    b History of previous blood transfusions
    c Jaundiced babies in earlier pregnancies

2 Investigations:
    a Rh-screening in all pregnancies
    b Check Rh-negative mothers for antibody titre and do indirect Coombs testing at regular intervals during pregnancy. Severe disease is rarely seen when the antibody titre is 1:16 or less
    c Amniocentesis is performed on any Rh-negative woman with a high antibody titre (greater than 1:16) or with a history of previous Rh-haemolytic disease. Elevated levels of bilirubin and its metabolites are detected by sequential optical density measurements of amniotic fluid. These may reveal three groups of fetus:
        i Unaffected
        ii Mild – may need exchange transfusion

　　iii Severe – needs exchange transfusions until
　　　　delivery can be effected at around 37 weeks
d Check baby immediately after delivery, and take
　umbilical cord blood for:
　i ABO grouping
　ii Rh grouping
　iii Indirect Coombs testing
　iv Full blood count
　v Bilirubin baseline level

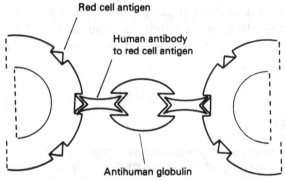

Figure 9.2 *Diagrammatic representation of the Coombs test*

The Coombs' test (antiglobulin reaction) (Figure 9.2): This detects adsorbed antibodies on the surface of erythrocytes. It uses either the patient's own red cells ('Direct' test) or normal red cells previously mixed with the patient's serum ('Indirect' test). Anti-human globulin is then added to the red cell suspension. The antiglobulin reacts with the antibody attached to the red cells and causes agglutination. Thus antiglobulin added to a suspension of fetal red cells will produce agglutination if maternal Rh antibody is attached to these cells.

Clinical features

Jaundice occurring within the first 24 h of life is usually caused by rhesus haemolytic disease.

1 Features due to elevated bilirubin levels:
  a Clinical jaundice
  b Kernicterus – bilirubin deposition in the brain particularly in the basal ganglia
2 Features due to red cell haemolysis:
  Classification:
  a Haemolytic anaemia of the newborn:
      i Haemoglobin level 12–16 g/100 ml (NR 16–18)
      ii Jaundice usually absent
      iii Good prognosis
  b Erythroblastosis fetalis (haemolytic disease of the newborn):
      i High peripheral reticulocyte count
      ii Due to increased manufacture of red blood cells in:
        • Bone marrow
        • Liver and spleen ('extramedullary haemopoiesis')
  c Hydrops fetalis:
      i Cause: Haemolytic process outstripping capacity of red cell producing organs to counteract the anaemia
      ii Clinical features ('Buddha in the uterus'):
        • Fetal heart failure
        • Generalized fetal anaemia
        • Ascites and pleural effusion
        • Hepatosplenomegaly
        • Usually ends in intrauterine death

Prevention

This has been possible since the mid-1960s. Give 50–100 μg anti-D gamma-globulin to all Rh-negative women in the presence of a positive indirect Coombs test (see above):

1　After delivery of all Rh-positive babies, as found from a test specimen of umbilical cord blood

2　After abortions

Anti-D globulin is about 98% effective in preventing Rh iso-immunization; its mechanism of action is unknown; but it is thought that anti-D globulin coats the fetal cells and unites with and neutralizes the D-factor

Treatment

1　Intrauterine transfusion of Rh-negative red cells, usually after the 25th week and before the 33rd week of gestation

2　Appropriate timing of the induction of labour. Premature delivery around the 35th–36th week of gestation may be necessary in some cases

3　Treat jaundice as appropriate (see below)

4　Treatment of hydrops fetalis: by exchange transfusion using twice the infant's calculated blood volume

NB: The perinatal mortality due to Rh disease has dropped from 45% in the 1940s to about 5% in the 1970s

HAEMOLYTIC DISEASE DUE TO ABO INCOMPATIBILITY

Incidence:

1　Approximately 1 in 200 deliveries

2　Girls more frequently affected

3　Can occur in the first child

Pathophysiology: The commonest occurrence is when the mother has blood group O, and the fetus has blood group A or B:

1   Normally the anti-A and Anti-B present in the mother's blood is entirely IgM and is not able to cross the placenta

2   However in certain cases the antibody may be present as an IgG. This can cross the placenta and cause a mild haemolytic disease

Diagnosis:
1   Coombs test – usually negative or only weakly positive

2   Mother blood group O and baby with blood group A or B

3   Prominent spherocytosis in fetal blood

Management: Haemolytic disease usually mild: photo-therapy usually suffices

NB: Other antibodies such as Kell, Duffy and MNS anti-bodies may cause haemolytic disease and all pregnant women should be screened for these antibodies at their first antenatal visit

Some differences between Rhesus and ABO incompatibility

	Rhesus	ABO
Prediction from antenatal testing	Yes	Not practicable
First infant affected	Rarely	Often
Subsequent infants affected	Yes	Affected randomly
Direct Coombs test (infant's red cells)	Positive	Negative or weakly positive
Intrauterine death	Can occur	Rarely
Anaemia at delivery	Common	Rare
Severity of jaundice	Variable: from mild to severe	Usually mild

TREATMENT OF NEONATAL JAUNDICE

1 Prevention: reduction of the incidence of pre-term delivery

2 Investigation for, and correction of, the underlying condition

3 Treatment of the hyperbilirubinaemia
   a Phototherapy:
      i Increases oxidative decomposition of bilirubin (to bilirubin E) in the skin
      ii Indicated where serum bilirubin reaches 170 μmol/l
      iii Bilirubin E does not cause brain cell damage
      Side-effects of phototherapy include diarrhoea, skin rashes, unstable thermoregulation, retinal damage, mild dehydration and 'bronzing'.
   b Enzyme induction: Administration of phenobarbitone induces synthesis of glucuronyl transferase in the liver. This is only indicated in some cases of Crigler–Najjar syndrome
   c Albumin infusion: 1 g/kg body weight in some infants to boost bilirubin binding capacity – rarely used
   d Exchange transfusion (used only in severely affected infants):
      i Removal of bilirubin containing blood and its replacement by healthy donor blood. Indicated if unconjugated bilirubin exceeds 340 μmol/l (20 mg%) and/or
      ii Replacing blood of low haematocrit with blood of high haematocrit in treating neonatal anaemic disease
      iii Objective is to correct anaemia, stop haemolysis and prevent a rise in bilirubin bound to albumin

Side-effects of exchange transfusion:
- Infection
- Embolization
- Anaemia
- Haemorrhage
- Necrotizing enterocolitis
- Convulsions
- Arrhythmias
- Cardiac arrest
- Hypoglycaemia
- Hypocalcaemia
- Hyperkalaemia
- Acidaemia

Jaundice in the premature infant

Pre-term infants are especially at risk from bilirubin toxicity, and kernicterus may result in pre-term infants with unconjugated bilirubin levels even as low as 12 mg% (200 μmol/l). This is due to the following:

1 Pre-term infants are more likely to experience cold stress. This causes the release of free fatty acids that displace bilirubin from albumin, its protein carrier

2 Pre-term infancy is associated with acidosis due to more common respiratory disorders. This also displaces bilirubin from albumin

3 Pre-term infants may have lower activities of glucuronyl transferase in the liver, and also lower absolute amounts of this enzyme

HAEMATOLOGICAL DISORDERS

Pallor

This is a serious sign and requires prompt management. The normal term infant is pale pink.

Pallor of rapid onset. This may be due to:

1 Haemolysis due to
  a Haemolytic disease
  b Severe infection

2 Circulatory collapse

3 Blood loss: this may be:
  a Before/during delivery:
    i Rupture of placental vessels due to placenta praevia
    ii Fetomaternal transfusion
  b After delivery:
    i External blood loss: from umbilical cord, gastrointestinal tract or injury
    ii Internal blood loss: haemorrhage into brain, lung or adrenals carries a poor prognosis

Pallor of gradual onset: This most frequently results, in pre-term infants, from a progressive fall in haemoglobin due to bone marrow inactivity

Anaemia

This may be due to:

1 Fetal haemorrhage
2 Feto-maternal transfusion
3 Feto-placental transfusion at delivery
4 Fetal haemolytic disease
5 Neonatal haemorrhage

Bleeding disorders

1 Vitamin K deficiency: Bacteria from the intestine normally produce sufficient vitamin K, but in the newborn the bowel is incompletely colonized by bacteria (vitamin K is involved in the production of

clotting factors II, VII, IX, X). Vitamin K deficiency is found in:
  a Premature infants
  b Infants receiving antibiotics
  c Mothers taking drugs that interfere with the effect of vitamin K on the synthesis of clotting factors, e.g. phenytoin, phenobarbitone, and salicylates

2 Haemorrhagic disease of newborn:
Pathophysiology: A haemorrhagic diathesis in newborn infants deficient in vitamin-K-dependent factors

Clinical features:
  a Generalized bleeding tendency within first 3 days
  b Prothrombin time and partial thromboplastin time prolonged

Management: 1–2 mg vitamin K. Bleeding stops in 6–12 h. If haemorrhage is life-threatening, fresh plasma or fresh whole blood transfusion (10 ml/kg) produces immediate results

Prevention: Since disorder can be prevented by administration of vitamin K, it should be given prophylactically to all newborn infants (1 mg intramuscularly)

3 Disturbances of clotting, e.g. disseminated intravascular coagulation (DIC), which may be caused by:
  a Septicaemia
  b Shock
  c Tissue release of thromboplastins: placenta abruptio, respiratory distress syndrome and hypoxia
  d Necrotizing enterocolitis
  e Renal vein thrombosis

4 Platelet disorders:
  a Maternal idiopathic thrombocytopenia
  b Maternal disseminated lupus erythematosus
  c Infants of mothers who received drugs such as quinine, digitalis and sulphonamides
  d Prenatal infectious disorders – 'TORCH' and postnatal infections (see page 71)
  e Disseminated intravascular coagulation (DIC)
  f Giant haemangioma – Kassabach's syndrome
  g Leukaemia and marrow hypoplasia

5 Inherited disorders:
  a Sex-linked recessive (expressed in males):
    i Haemophilia – deficiency in the activity of clotting Factor VIII
    ii Christmas disease – deficiency of clotting Factor IX
  b Autosomal dominant:
    i Von Willebrands' disease – deficiency of clotting factor VIII and an impairment of platelet function
  c Autosomal recessive: Deficiency of:
    i Fibrinogen (Factor I)
    ii Prothrombin (Factor II)
    iii Factors V, VII, X, XII and XIII

10

Infection

The incidence, mortality and morbidity of neonatal infections is considerably lower than it was at the turn of the century.

Routes of infection

1 Transplacental: from maternal blood via the placenta	Intrauterine infection: Clinical manifestations often present at birth
2 Ascending: premature rupture of membranes allowing infections via maternal vagina	
3 Intrapartum: acquired during passage through birth canal	Extrauterine infection: clinical manifestations present more than 1 day after birth
4 Postnatal: organisms acquired from environment after birth	

Defence mechanisms against infection:
1 Passive immunity – transfer of maternal immunoglobin G (IgG) from the mother in the last trimester
2 Fetal immunoglobin M (IgM) may be present if previous intrauterine infection occurred

143

3 Serum complement

4 Lysozymes and lactoferrin, particularly in mother's milk

5 Fetal blood leukocytes – but phagocytosis is inefficient in the newborn

Risk groups for intrauterine fetal infection

1 Unexplained maternal illness during pregnancy: particularly appearance of a fever or rash

2 Membrane rupture/delivery interval exceeding 24 h

3 Maternal pyrexia immediately before, during, or after labour

4 Abnormal maternal vaginal discharge immediately before, during, or after labour

5 Small-for-dates fetus

General clinical features of neonatal infection

1 'Failure to thrive'

2 Diarrhoea and vomiting

3 Irritability

4 Apnoeic attacks

5 Hypoglycaemia

6 Jaundice

7 Unstable thermoregulation – hypothermia or hyperthermia

8 Splenomegaly and hepatomegaly

9 Purpuric skin rash

10 Often small-for-dates

TRANSPLACENTAL INFECTION

1 Non-bacterial infections:
   a Cytomegalovirus

    b Toxoplasmosis
    c Rubella
2 Bacterial:
    a *Treponema pallidum* (Syphilis)
    b *Mycobacterium tuberculosis*
    c *Listeria monocytogenes*

Cytomegalovirus

Incidence: 1 in 200 of all pregnancies

Clinical consequences:
1 Most cases are asymptomatic or mild
2 Full clinical picture may produce:
    a Early jaundice
    b Purpura
    c Haemolytic anaemia
    d Hepatosplenomegaly
    e Pneumonia with cough
    f Fits
    g Microcephaly
    h Chorioretinitis
    i Cataract
    j Congenital heart disease
3 Infection in the 1st trimester is associated with:
    a Abortion
    b Stillbirth
    c Premature delivery
    d 'Small-for-dates' fetus
4 Congenital cytomegalovirus infection in the newborn may:
    a Be asymptomatic
    b Show features of acute manifestation of infection (see list above)
    c Cause excretion of virus in urine for several years

5 Long-term sequelae of symptomatic viral infection include:
  a Microcephaly
  b Mental and motor retardation

Investigation of cytomegalovirus infection:
1 Of the mother:
  a Isolation of virus from cervical swabs and urine
  b Serological detection using IgM-specific antibody
2 Of the child:
  a Isolation of the virus from nasopharynx, conjunctivae, urine ('owl's-eye cells') and cerebrospinal fluid
  b Serological detection uses IgM-specific antibody. This is less sensitive

Management of cytomegalovirus infection:
1 In the mother
  a No specific treatment if asymptomatic
  b Symptomatic treatment if mononucleosis-like illness is present
2 In the child: Most cases are asymptomatic. No satisfactory specific measures are available but highly infectious cases should be barrier-nursed

Toxoplasmosis

Toxoplasma gondii is a protozoon. The route of transmission to pregnant women is thought to be through meat and cat faeces

Incidence: About 0.07% of all pregnancies

Clinical features:
1 In the mother: Occasionally lymphadenopathy – usually asymptomatic

2 In the child: Similar to cytomegalovirus

Management:
1 Mother:
  a No preventive vaccine available
  b Avoid known sources of toxoplasma
2 Child: Consider use of pyrimethamine and other anti-
  protozoal agents

Rubella

Incidence: 0.1–2.5% pregnancies. Of these, 0.07–0.7%
will result in congenital abnormalities

Clinical consequences: Risk of congenital malformations
associated with infection even up to 24th week of gestation.
High rate of abortion if acute infection occurs in 1st month
of gestation

Clinical features of rubella:
1 In the mother:
  a History of exposure 2–3 weeks previously
  b '3-day rash' of pink-red maculopapules
  c Mild fever, headache, malaise, lymphadeno-
    pathy and joint pains

2 In the child:
  a Bone abnormalities
  b Microcephaly and mental retardation
  c Deafness
  d Eyes: cataracts, glaucoma, retinitis
  e Heart: cardiac defects including pulmonary
    stenosis, patent ductus arteriosus, ventricular
    septal defect and congenital myocarditis
  f Hepatosplenomegaly with or without jaundice.

Investigations:
1 In the mother:
   a Specific rubella antibody (IgM) test
   b Antibody seroconversion tests
2 In the infant:
   a Elevated antibody titre for up to 3 months
   b Virus isolation from throat or urine

Management of rubella:
1 Mother:
   a Mild analgesia
   b Document infection by serial serological testing
2 Child:
   a Isolate: virus may be shed from nasopharynx for as long as 12 months
   b Clinical investigations for congenital malformation

Prevention:
Rubella antibody titre to identify women at risk during pregnancy
1 A negative or low titre suggests susceptibility to the disease
2 A high titre suggests immunity
3 A rising titre suggests a recent active infection

Live attenuated vaccine is given to schoolgirls aged 10–13 and seronegative postpartum women. In the USA vaccination against rubella is given to young children. Approximately 15% of American women of child-bearing age remain susceptible to rubella

ASCENDING INFECTION

Pathophysiology:
1 Premature rupture of membranes may allow organisms in the maternal vagina to enter the amniotic cavity and be inhaled by the fetus

2 Causative organisms include *Staphylococcus aureus*, Streptococci, *E. coli*, *Bacillus proteus*, *Listeria monocytogenes* and *Candida albicans*

Clinical features:
1 Diffuse pneumonia. May be indistinguishable from respiratory distress syndrome in infections with β-haemolytic streptococci
2 Lethargy, vomiting, cyanosis
3 Weight loss and failure to thrive
4 Death may occur before delivery

Treatment:
Antibiotic therapy after testing amniotic fluid

INTRAPARTUM INFECTION

Pathophysiology:
1 Infection acquired during passage of fetus through the birth canal
2 Organisms include: Streptococci, *E. coli*, *Candida albicans*, *Listeria monocytogenes*, *Neisseria gonorrhoeae*, *Mycoplasma pneumoniae*, *Herpes simplex*

Clinical examples:
1 *Listeria monocytogenes*
   a Septicaemia and meningitis
   b Usually treated with ampicillin
2 Group B streptococci:
   a Bacteraemia with meningitis or cyanosis and/or respiratory distress syndrome
   b Treated with penicillin
3 Gonorrhoea: Ophthalmia neonatorum:
   a Severe purulent conjunctivitis caused by infection of the conjunctival sac

    b Treat with local and systemic penicillin

NB: The commonest causative organisms in ophthalmia neonatorum are *Staphylococcus aureus* and *Bacillus proteus*. Gonococcal ophthalmia may lead to blindness and must be treated vigorously

Neisseria

Pathophysiology: This is acquired when the fetus passes through the birth canal, and the infection typically begins in the neonate as a purulent conjunctivitis. This may lead to corneal perforation with blindness if left untreated.

Clinical features:
1 In the mother:
    a Many cases are asymptomatic
    b In a few cases, one or more of the following may occur:
        i Pelvic peritonitis
        ii Premature membrane rupture
        iii Chorioamnionitis
        iv Septic polyarthritis

2 In the child:
    a Unexplained sepsis
    b Purulent conjunctivitis (ophthalmia neonatorum)
    c Septic polyarthritis
    d Meningitis

Investigation of gonorrhoea:
1 Of the mother
    a Vaginal swabs with cultures as indicated by the history of sexual exposure
    b Blood culture

2 Of the child:
    a Microscopy using Gram staining of conjunctival swab reveals Gram-negative intracellular diplococci

b Eye, blood and lumbar puncture cultures may be positive for gonococci

Management of gonorrhoea:
1 For the mother (subject to antibiotic sensitivity in the patient):
  a Asymptomatic, localized infection: Procaine penicillin G 5 megaunits i.m. and probenecid 1 g orally
  b Systemic infection: 10 megaunits i.m. penicillin daily for 10–14 days
2 For the child:
  a Ophthalmia neonatorum: Penicillin drops in both eyes (10 000 units/ml) and 0.05 megaunits kg^{-1} day^{-1} for 7 days. Ophthalmological advice should be sought
  b Systemic infection: 75 000–100 000 units kg^{-1} day^{-1} for 7 days of penicillin

NB: Reports of penicillinase-producing strains of *Neisseria gonorrhoeae* necessitate full culture and sensitivity and close follow-up

Herpes infection

Pathophysiology: Caused by herpes simplex type I (HSV-1) or II (HSV-2) acquired at the time of vaginal delivery. HSV-2 is implicated in 80–90% of cases.

Clinical features:
1 In the mother:
  a Herpetic lesions occur on cervix, vagina and genital area
  b Lymphadenopathy
2 In the infant: three general types of presentation:
  a Localized – 15% of cases: Herpetic lesions occur on eyes, oral cavity and skin

    b Central nervous system – 15% of cases:
       i Localized lesions may be present
      ii Lethargy, anorexia, vomiting, irritability
    c Disseminated – 70% of cases
       i Features of severe systemic infection – jaundice, purpura, shock
      ii CNS and localized involvements may also be present

Investigation:
1 Of the mother:
    a Direct isolation of virus – this is the most sensitive and specific
    b Indirect detection of virus by immunological tests is less sensitive. In addition many 'normal' individuals may have HSV-1 or HSV-2 antibody
2 Of the child:
    a Isolation of the virus from vesicle fluid, nasopharynx, urine and cerebrospinal fluid – this is the most sensitive test
    b Serological tests: Antibody in CSF or blood

Prevention of HSV infection:
1 During pregnancy: Avoid sexual contact with consort with herpetic lesion
2 Delivery: Deliver by Caesarean section before membrane rupture if virus or lesions are present in the last 2 weeks of pregnancy
3 After delivery: Isolate infected infant. Appropriate hygiene precautions for parents

Management: Treatment with either adenosine arabinoside or 5-iodo-2-deoxyuridine (idoxuridine) and gamma globulin if there are systemic manifestations. Mortality can be as high as 60%

Hepatitis B

Pathophysiology: Hepatitis B antigen is present in about 0.1% of adults in Europe and the USA, and 5–15% of adults in South-East Asia. The hepatitis B virus may be transmitted to the infant either during the pregnancy if infection occurs towards the time of delivery or in the postpartum period

Clinical features:
1 In the mother:
    a History of exposure between 60 and 200 days previously
    b Pyrexia, dark urine, jaundice and liver enlargement
2 In the child:
    a Usually asymptomatic
    b 10% may become jaundiced

Investigations:
1 In the mother:
    a Increase in serum transaminases and abnormal liver function tests
    b Presence of hepatitis B surface antigen (HB_sAg) in blood
    Presence of hepatitis B_e antigen (HB_eAg) in blood implies an increased risk of transmission of disease to the infant
2 In the child:
    a Persistent HB_sAg in serum
    b Liver biopsy may remain abnormal for many months

Prevention:
1 In the mother:
    a Minimize exposure to hepatitis
    b Administer hepatitis B immune globulin (HBIG)

or immune serum globulin (ISG) if HBIG is not available

2   In the child: If mother has hepatitis B during pregnancy and is HB$_s$Ag-positive at term, administer HBIG (or ISG) on the day of birth

Management of hepatitis B:
1   In the mother:
   a   Rest and symptomatic treatment
   b   High-protein and low-fat diet
   c   Sterile precautions, especially with use of hypodermic needles
2   In the child:
   a   Rest and symptomatic treatment
   b   No specific treatment
   c   Sterile precautions

POSTNATAL INFECTION

Aetiology and pathophysiology:
1   Failure of preventive measures against infection with failure of infant's resistance to infection
2   Organisms involved:
   a   Gram-positive organisms
     Examples: Staphylococci, pyogenic Streptococci
     Clinical features:
       i   First clinical signs usually superficial – redness, swelling. Production of pus
      ii   More widespread haematogenous spread may follow
   b   Gram-negative organisms: Widespread infection with bacteraemia, urinary tract infection and meningitis

Clinical features:
1   Superficial infection:
   a   Infant usually not systemically ill

  b Greater risks of cross infection
   Examples:
   i Conjunctivitis
   ii Pustules
   iii Impetigo
   iv Paronychia
   v Umbilical stump infection
   vi Thrush – commonly affects the mouth but
    may also involve the oesophagus and gastro-
    intestinal tract

2 'Deep' infection. Generalized systemic illness:
 a Inactivity
 b Feeding difficulty
 c Weight loss
 d Pallor
 e Cyanosis and dyspnoea – usually late signs
 f Jaundice
 g Irritability
 h Vomiting
 i Ileus
 Poor prognosis

Investigation of neonatal infections

1 Culture and microscopy of:
 a Urine
 b Cerebrospinal fluid
 c Stools
 d Amniotic fluid
 e Maternal vaginal swab
 f Gastric aspirate
2 Culture of:
 a Throat swab
 b Nose and ear swabs
 c Blood culture
 d Umbilical swab

3   Haematology: Blood film and white cell count of cord and baby's blood

4   Serology: Serum IgM and particular antibodies as indicated for both cord and baby's blood

5   Radiology: Chest and abdominal X-ray

6   Histology and culture of placenta

7   Blood gases

Management

Prevention:
1   Feed babies with fresh human milk; this has antibacterial properties

2   Scrupulous handwashing before and after handling each baby

3   Use of aseptic techniques in particular procedures, e.g. intubation, catheterization, etc.

4   Sterilization of equipment, e.g. incubators, washbasins, sinks, etc.

5   Early diagnosis and treatment of neonatal infection, to reduce incidence of cross-infection

Treatment:
1   Begin treatment immediately after specimens are taken with broad-spectrum antibiotics. Therapy may be modified in the light of bacterial culture results

2   Intravenous fluids if needed to restore circulation and correct any coexistent metabolic disorders

3   Investigation and treatment of any haemorrhage

4   Intensive therapy in a special-care baby unit may be necessary

11

Metabolic Problems

Problems of infants of diabetic mothers

1 Respiratory distress
2 Hypoglycaemia
3 Hypocalcaemia
4 Hyperbilirubinaemia
5 Congestive heart failure
6 Congenital malformations
7 Polycythaemia
8 Renal vein thrombosis
9 Hypercoagulability
10 Sepsis
11 Prematurity

Hypoglycaemia (blood glucose less than about 1.4 mmol/l (25 mg/dl))

High risk situations:
1 'Light-for-dates' babies (deficient glycogen stores)
2 Infants of diabetic mothers (fetal hyperinsulinism)
3 Haemolytic disease of the newborn

4 Respiratory distress syndrome

5 Hypothermia and cold injury

6 Asphyxia and sepsis

7 Inherited metabolic disorders

Clinical features:
1 Many infants are asymptomatic

2 Irritability and pallor

3 Reluctance to feed and listlessness

4 Twitching and convulsions

5 Temperature instability

Treatment:
1 Prevention: with early frequent feeding

2 If mild: frequent feeds with added glucose (5%) or increased milk feeds

3 If severe: 10% glucose given intravenously, slowly by scalp or limb vein

4 If non-responsive to above give glucagon or ACTH

Prognosis: Can lead to brain damage if convulsions not treated

Hypocalcaemia

Serum calcium below 1.8 mmol/l (7 mg/dl). May cause tetany of the newborn

Aetiology:
1 Hypocalcaemia occurring during the first 3 days after birth:
  a Maternal causes:
    i Diabetes mellitus
    ii Pre-eclampsia and eclampsia

   iii Hyperparathyroidism or a dietary lack of calcium
 b Intrapartum causes:
     i Prematurity
     ii Asphyxia
 c Postnatal causes:
     i Respiratory distress syndrome
     ii Hypoxia
     iii Shock
     iv Sepsis
     v Metabolic acidosis
2 Hypocalcaemia occurring after the first three days (rarer):
 a Bottle-fed babies – high phosphate diet (cow's milk)
 b Vitamin D deficiency
 c Hypoparathyroidism
 d Renal disease

Clinical features:
1 Local twitchings of limbs
2 Generalized convulsions
3 Apnoeic spells and cyanosis
4 Laryngospasm or carpopedal spasm

Treatment: Oral or parenteral calcium supplementation (calcium gluconate) and vitamin D

Prognosis: Good – long-term sequelae rare

Metabolic acidosis (see also Chapter 16)

Occurrence: This is an end-event from any factor that results in a compromised delivery of oxygen to tissues. It may occur in association with the following causes:
1 Fetal distress

2 Neonatal asphyxia

3 Shock and hypovolaemia

4 Neonatal sepsis

5 Intracranial haemorrhage

6 Necrotizing enterocolitis

7 Renal tubular acidosis

8 Cardiorespiratory disorders that result in decreased arterial oxygen pressures

Clinical features. These may include:
1 History of prolonged resuscitation in the delivery room
2 Tachypnoea
3 Features of the underlying cause

Investigations. An arterial blood gas sample will reveal:
1 PCO_2 is either:
   a On the low side of normal in uncompensated metabolic acidosis
   b Low, in compensated metabolic acidosis
2 pH is either:
   a Low, in uncompensated metabolic acidosis, or
   b Normal in compensated metabolic acidosis

Management:
1 Correction of the underlying cause
2 Correction of the base deficit (see Chapter 16)

Other electrolyte disorders – see Chapter 16

Inborn errors of metabolism

There are an enormous number of genetically transmitted disorders, the majority of which are very rare and involve a deficiency of a single enzyme. They are usually autosomal recessives and need not cause symptoms in the neonatal period

A MAJOR CLINICAL FEATURES MAY INCLUDE:
1 Feeding difficulties or vomiting

2 Seizures

3 Jaundice

4 Hepatomegaly

5 Hypoglycaemia

6 Metabolic acidosis

7 Ketosis

8 Hyperammonaemia

9 Abnormal odour to sweat or urine

10 Coarse facial features

11 Reducing substances in the urine

12 Positive ferric chloride reaction in the urine

B LIST OF INBORN ERRORS OF METABOLISM PRESENTING IN THE NEONATAL PERIOD
1 Carbohydrate metabolism
  a Galactosaemia (galactose-1-phosphate uridyl transferase deficiency)
  b Hereditary fructose intolerance (fructose-1-phosphate aldolase deficiency)
  c Fructose-1,6-diphosphatase deficiency
  d Glycogen storage disease, type I (von Gierke's disease, glucose-6-phosphatase deficiency)
  e Glycogen storage disease, type II (Pompe's disease, α-1,4-glucosidase deficiency)
  f Glycogen storage disease, type III (limit dextrinosis, debrancher deficiency)
  g Glycogen storage disease, type IV (amylopectinosis, brancher deficiency)
2 Mucopolysaccharide metabolism
  a Hurler syndrome (mucopolysaccharidosis I, alpha-L-iduronidase deficiency)

    b Hunter syndrome (mucopolysaccharidosis II, iduronosulfate deficiency)

    c β-Glucuronidase deficiency

3 Disorders of lipid metabolism

    a GM_1 gangliosidosis, type I (generalized gangliosidosis, β-galactosidase deficiency)

    b GM_3 gangliosidosis

    c Wolman's disease (acid lipase deficiency)

    d Niemann–Pick disease, types A and B (sphingomyelinase deficiency)

4 Amino acid metabolism or transport

    a Maple syrup urine disease

    b Hypervalinaemia

    c Hyperlysinaemia

    d Hyper-β-alaninaemia

    e Non-ketotic hyperglycinaemia

    f Phenylketonuria

    g Oasthouse urine disease (methionine malabsorption)

    h Tyrosinaemia

    i Hypermethioninaemia

    j Homocystinuria

    k Hartnup disease

5 Urea cycle defects

    a Carbamylphosphate synthetase deficiency (hyperammonaemia type I)

    b Ornithine transcarbamylase deficiency (hyperammonaemia type II)

    c Citrullinaemia

    d Argininosuccinic aciduria

    e Arginase deficiency

6 Organic acid metabolism

    a Methylmalonic acidaemia

    b Propionic acidaemia (ketotic hyperglycinaemia)

    c Isovaleric acidaemia

    d Butyric and hexanoic acidaemia

    e β-Methylcrotonyl–CoA carboxylase deficiency

7 Other disorders

    a Adrenogenital syndrome

    b Lysosomal acid phosphate deficiency

    c Renal tubular acidosis

    d Nephrogenic diabetes insipidus

    e Menke's kinky hair syndrome

    f Orotic aciduria

    g Congenital lactic acidosis

    h Cystic fibrosis

i Hypophosphatasia
j Fucosidosis
k Crigler–Najjar syndrome
l α_1-Antitrypsin deficiency
m I-cell disease (mucolipidosis II)
n Albinism
o Lesch–Nyhan syndrome

Phenylketonuria

Elevated plasma phenylalanine levels due to diminished conversion of phenylalanine to tyrosine. This is an autosomal recessive disorder

Incidence: 1:10 000 to 1:20 000 live births

Aetiology: Absence of liver enzyme phenylalanine hydroxylase leads to accumulation of phenylalanine in plasma. Vomiting is often the only resulting symptom in the first months of life

Clinical features of phenylketonuria in an untreated child:

1 Severe mental retardation

2 Usually blond with blue eyes

3 Hyperactivity, psychosis

4 Convulsions and marked EEG abnormalities

5 Unpleasant body odour in child or a parent

Management: Dietary restriction of phenylalanine and regular blood phenylalanine checks

Recognition of phenylketonuria, galactosaemia and maple syrup urine disease uses the Guthrie test. The Guthrie inhibition assay test requires only a few drops of capillary blood. Inhibition of growth of a bacterial culture provides the diagnosis but this if positive is urgently confirmed by further biochemical tests.

Galactosaemia

Incidence: 1 in 40 000 to 1 in 60 000. An inborn error of carbohydrate metabolism in which galactose-1-phosphate cannot be converted to glucose-1-phosphate. The infant is normal at birth, but within a few days there is jaundice, vomiting, diarrhoea, lethargy, hypotonia and loss of weight. Liver damage and cataracts may also result. It is managed by limiting dietary lactose and galactose.

C SOME INBORN ERRORS OF METABOLISM WHICH MAY BE LETHAL IN NEONATES.
Most are autosomal recessives

Disease	Methods of detection
Carbamyl phosphate synthetase deficiency	Blood ammonia
Ornithine transcarbamylase deficiency (X-linked)	Blood ammonia
Citrullinaemia	Blood ammonia, HVE* of urine or serum
Other forms of hyperammonaemia	Blood ammonia
Propionic acidaemia	Metabolic acidosis, GLC† of urine
Methylmalonic acidaemia	Metabolic acidosis, GLC of urine
Maple syrup urine disease	Metabolic acidosis, HVE of urine or serum, GLC of urine
Isovaleric acidaemia	Metabolic acidosis, GLC of urine
Non-ketotic hyperglycinaemia	Clinical features, HVE of urine and serum
Galactosaemia	Clinical features, glycosuria
Hereditary fructose intolerance	Clinical features, glycosuria
Hereditary tyrosinaemia	Clinical features, HVE of urine and serum, GLC of urine
Pyridoxine-dependent convulsions	Clinical features, therapeutic response
Congenital lactic acidosis	Metabolic acidosis, GLC of urine

*HVE = high voltage electrophoresis
†GLC = gas−liquid chromatography

D MANAGEMENT OF INFANTS WITH A SUSPECTED METABOLIC DISORDER
Remember that the odds are three to one that the baby is normal

1 Delivery at term except when spontaneous premature labour occurs

2 Baby is transferred to a specialized metabolic unit after delivery and assessed by a paediatrician

3 Blood tests for:
   a Glucose
   b pH, HCO_3^-
   c Ketones
   d Amino acids
   e Potassium and sodium
   f Ammonia
   g Organic acids
   h Calcium and magnesium

4 Urine examination:
   a Colour
   b Odour
   c Sediment
   d Ketone
   e Reaction to ferric chloride
   f Amino acids

5 If a metabolic disturbance is demonstrated, management is determined by the diagnosis

12

Neurological Problems

CONGENITAL ABNORMALITIES OF THE NERVOUS SYSTEM

The most serious such as anencephaly, encephalocoele and spina bifida develop in the first 2 months of gestation.

1 Anencephaly: This is an absence of cranial vault bones and cerebral hemispheres. The death rate is 100%, most infants dying during delivery or stillborn. Antenatal diagnosis:
   a Abdominal palpation
   b Hydramnios
   c Ultrasound studies
   d X-ray examination
   e Decreased oestrogen excretion
   f Raised amniotic maternal serum alpha-feto-protein (α FP) levels
   Treatment: Induce labour as soon as diagnosed. Condition incompatible with life.

2 Microcephaly: Infants have small heads and severe mental retardation. May occur in association with intrauterine infections, e.g. rubella.

3 Hydrocephaly: Excessive accumulation of CSF within the ventricles causing head enlargement. May be

caused by obstruction to CSF flow within ventricular channels, particularly at the foramina of Luschka and Magendie, in the roof of the fourth ventricle. Hydrocephaly can also be caused by excessive production and/or impaired absorption of CSF. Communicating hydrocephalus is present when the CSF flows freely into the subarachnoid space. Non-communicating hydrocephalus indicates no free flow of CSF.

Antenatal diagnosis:

a   Large head on palpation
b   Hydramnios
c   Ultrasound studies
d   Radiological studies – separation of sutures, bulging fontanelles and a 'copper-beaten' skull.

Treatment: Gross hydrocephaly is not treated. Cerebrospinal fluid can be shunted by catheter from the lateral ventricle to neck veins, the peritoneal cavity or the right atrium, to by-pass the site of blockage. This is achieved by use of a by-pass valve of the

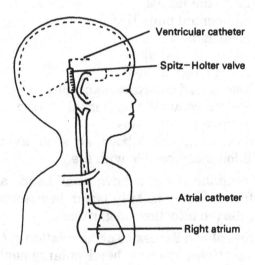

Figure 12.1   *Diagram of ventriculo-atrial drainage incorporating a Spitz–Holter valve*

Spitz–Holter type that shunts fluid from the ventricle to the right atrium (Figure 12.1).

Prognosis: Mortality 50% if untreated. Mental retardation and physical handicaps are common.

4 Spina bifida (Figure 12.2): Spina bifida usually occurs in the lumbar, low thoracic or sacral region and extends for about 3–6 vertebral segments. The fault is a mesodermal defect causing failure of fusion of vertebral arches of one or more vertebrae. Herniation of the meninges or spinal cord may result.

There are both genetic and environmental factors in the aetiology of spina bifida. It is commonest in first-born.

Treatment: Where there is a defect, cover with sterile material and consider surgical closure. Infection leading to meningitis may supervene. Most paediatricians and surgeons only recommend surgery in about 25% of these infants. The selection is based

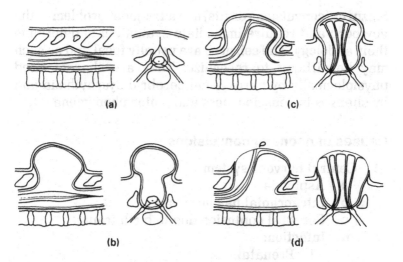

(a)

(c)

(b)

(d)

Figure 12.2 *Spina bifida: (a) spina bifida occulta;*
(b) meningocoele; (c) covered myelomeningocoele;
(d) open myelomeningocoele

Forms of spina bifida (see Figure 12.2):

	Bony arch	Skin	Meninges	Spinal cord
Spina bifida occulta	Defect	Hairy patch or dimple	Intact	Intact
Meningo-coele	Defect	Intact	Intact but bulging	Intact
Meningo-myelocoele	Defect	Defect	Bulge to surface	Some involvement. Possible sphincter paralysis
Myelocoele	Defect	Defect	Defect	Defective and exposed to surface

upon the outlook for survival and the future quality of life and amount of functioning nervous system.

Prognosis: Good with simple meningocoele if closed surgically.

NEONATAL CONVULSIONS

Seizures (convulsions or fits) are a frequent problem in the newborn and require immediate evaluation to determine their aetiology. The seizures are usually focal and as such may be difficult to recognize. They are characterized physiologically by paroxysmal cerebral dysrhythmia and by changes in consciousness and motor phenomena

Causes of neonatal convulsions

1 Central nervous system:
    a Asphyxia
    b Intracranial haemorrhage
    c Cerebral contusion due to birth trauma
    d Infection:
        i Prenatal:
            • Rubella
            • Toxoplasmosis
            • Cytomegalovirus

    ii Meningitis: *E. coli, Listeria monocytogenes* and group B Streptococcus are the commonest pathogens causing pyogenic meningitis in the newborn
  e Kernicterus
  f Developmental abnormalities of the central nervous system

2 Metabolic:
  a Hypoglycaemia (blood glucose less than 1.5 mmol/l (25 mg/dl))
  b Hypocalcaemia
  c Hypomagnesaemia
  d Hyper- or hyponatraemia
  e Narcotic withdrawal
  f Inborn error of metabolism, e.g. maple syrup urine disease

3 Sepsis
Symptoms and signs: Because of the immaturity of the central nervous system the usual well-organized tonic–clonic seizure pattern may not be seen in the neonate
  a Lethargy, irritability and tremor
  b Eye-blinking, nystagmus
  c Variable body tone – hypotonia, spasticity
  d Apnoea with cyanosis and bradycardia
  e Colour changes and vasomotor disturbances

Investigation of convulsions

1 Full clinical examination including prenatal and natal history

2 Biochemical:
  a Serum calcium and phosphate
  b Blood urea nitrogen and creatinine
  c Blood sugar
  d Electrolytes

3 Haematological: white blood count ($>10\,000/mm^3$ implies infection)

4 Microbiological: If infection is suspected
  a Blood and other cultures
  b Viral screen
  c Urine analysis

5 Cerebrospinal fluid:
  a Lumbar puncture indicated if meningitis is suspected
  b Subdural tap as indicated

6 Skull X-ray

7 Electroencephalogram, in investigating origin of seizures

8 Brain and computerized axial tomography (CAT) may be indicated if a focal lesion is suspected. (6) and (7) are also indicated if there is a prolonged series of seizures

9 Brain biopsy if herpes encephalitis is suspected

Management

1 Nurse infant on side and clear the airway

2 Anticonvulsants such as phenobarbitone, paraldehyde, phenytoin, sodium valproate or diazepam for symptomatic control. Phenobarbitone and paraldehyde are the most commonly used; diazepam is used if these are not successful

3 Treat specific abnormality where indicated

4 Give oxygen in high concentration in incubator

Causes of a hyperactive baby

1 Low birth weight

2 Brain damage

3 Congenital thyrotoxicosis: This may occur in the off-spring in a mother with hyperthyroidism. It presents as a hyperactive baby with tachycardia, exophthalmos, and excessive appetite. It is managed with anti-thyroid drugs

4 Iatrogenic – for example secondary to doxapram therapy. Not common.

Causes of a drowsy baby

1 Normal variation

2 Pre-term baby

3 Cerebral injury due to hypoxia, mechanical trauma or cerebral haemorrhage

4 Increased intracranial pressure due to hydro-cephalus or haemorrhage

5 Infection

6 Hypothermia

7 Iatrogenic – sedation

8 Hypoglycaemia

Causes of a floppy baby

1 Cerebral malfunction
   a Subnormality
   b Birth trauma
   c Cerebral palsy

2 Hypoxia

3 Low birth weight

4 Rare causes: Include certain inborn errors of metabolism and neurological disorders

Conditions associated with mental defect

1   Chromosomal abnormalities:
    a   Down's syndrome (trisomy 21), occurs in 1:600 live births (see below)
    b   Trisomy D(13) (Patau's syndrome) and trisomy E(18) (Edwards' syndrome) are uncommon
    c   Cri-du-chat syndrome. Due to deletion of the short arms of chromosome S. Distinct facies and a peculiar cry resembling that of a cat
    d   Klinefelter's syndrome (XXY). See Chapter 5

2   Cranial abnormalities:
    a   Microcephaly: Cytomegalovirus or other intrauterine infections ('TORCH') are often responsible (see Chapter 10)
    b   Craniostenosis: Premature closure of one or other cranial sutures
    c   Hydrocephalus:
        i   Often associated with spina bifida
        ii Congenital toxoplasmosis is occasionally the cause

3   Maternal and fetal infections – 'TORCH' (see Chapter 10)

4   Biochemical causes:
    a   Genetic: Inborn errors of metabolism, e.g. phenylketonuria, galactosaemia, and congenital hypothyroidism. See Chapter 11
    b   Acquired
        i   Prenatal: drugs, and gross maternal metabolic disturbances, e.g. uncontrolled diabetes
        ii Neonatal and postnatal: poisoning, e.g. hypoxia, hypoglycaemia, carbon monoxide, heavy metals (e.g. lead and mercury)

5   Birth trauma

13

Gastrointestinal Problems

CONGENITAL ABNORMALITIES OF THE GASTROINTESTINAL SYSTEM

Cleft lip (hare lip) and cleft palate

Aetiology:
1 Genetic but complex
2 Exposure to anticonvulsant drugs in pregnancy
3 Associated with other malformations such as congenital heart anomalies
4 More frequent in males
5 Associated with many syndromes, e.g. Pierre–Robin

Embryology:
1 During the development of the face there are two maxillary processes which develop horizontally. These fuse with the frontal processes developing vertically. Thus failure of fusion on one or both sides results in unilateral or bilateral cleft lip respectively
2 Commoner in certain racial groups, e.g. Japanese

Clinical manifestations:
1 Cleft lip may vary from a small notch to a complete separation extending into the floor of the nose. Clefts

may be single or double. Main handicap is difficulty with feeding

2 Clefts of the palate may occur alone or in association with cleft lip. Isolated cleft palates occur in the midline

Management:
1 Feeding
   a Breast feeding is possible in cases of cleft lip alone or small clefts of the palate
   b Bottle feeding with large soft teat
   c Dental plate to occlude cleft or orthodontics

2 Operative repair of lip performed when baby is 3 months. Palate is left until 12–18 months – before speech commences

3 Orthodontics and speech care vitally important in later management

Oesophageal atresia

Often associated with tracheo-oesophageal fistula and other malformations (see also Chapter 5)

Diagnosis:
1 Hydramnios

2 Infant brings up frothy saliva

3 Abdomen distended with gas

4 Failure to pass a rubber nasogastric tube
Treatment: Early diagnosis is essential to avoid inhalation of feeds. Operation as soon as possible after birth
Prognosis: Usually good in treated cases

Pyloric stenosis

Hypertrophied pyloric muscle causing partial blockage of the pyloric lumen

Incidence: About 3:1000. Commoner in firstborn male infants; familial disorder

Clinical features: Usually manifest in 2nd and 3rd week of life but can be from 10 days to 10 weeks

1 Projectile vomiting occurring shortly after feeds

2 Weight loss despite a ravenous appetite

3 Visible gastric peristalsis

4 Constipation

5 Abdominal distension

6 Pyloric mass, especially demonstrable after test feeding.

Complications:

1 Dehydration

2 Metabolic alkalosis

3 Electrolyte imbalance

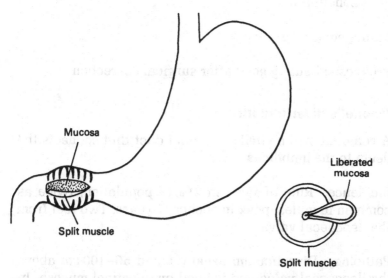

Figure 13.1 *Incision employed in pyloromyotomy (Ramstedt's operation) for pyloric stenosis. Inset shows mucosa protruding between cut edges of split muscle*

Management (Figure 13.1) Surgery to relieve obstruction – Ramstedt's operation – division of the hypertrophic pyloric muscles.

Prognosis: Usually good in treated cases

Duodenal, jejunal or ileal obstruction

Duodenal, jejunal or ileal obstruction may occur due to atresia (a complete blockage of the lumen). About 15% of intestinal atresias are multiple. Associated with Down's syndrome

Clinical manifestations:
1 History of hydramnios
2 Abdominal distension
3 Vomiting
4 Constipation

Management: Surgery

Prognosis: Usually good after surgical correction

Meckel's diverticulum

A remnant of the vitello-intestinal duct that connects the ileum to the umbilicus

Incidence: 'Rule of two': in 2% of population; twice as common in males; peak incidence, 2 years. Two feet from the ileocaecal valve

Pathology: Diverticulum usually found 50–100 cm above the ileocaecal valve and is lined by intestinal mucosa. In about 50% of cases there is also ectopic gastric, duodenal or pancreatic mucosa.

Clinical manifestations:

1 Symptoms occur most frequently before 2 years of age

2 Painless rectal bleeding usually without stool

3 Abdominal pain – clinical picture resembles appendicitis

4 Intussusception – Meckel's diverticulum may become the 'lead point' of an intussusception

5 Obstruction

6 Fistula formation

Complications:

1 Perforation with peritonitis

2 Haemorrhage

3 Bowel strangulation

4 Intussusception

5 Volvulus

6 Death

Management: Surgical excision of the diverticulum

Hirschsprung's disease

Congenital megacolon or intestinal aganglionosis

Incidence:

1 1:5000 with male dominance

2 Associated with Down's syndrome and abnormalities of the genitourinary system

Pathology: Absence of parasympathetic ganglion cells of Auerbach's and Meissner's plexuses in lower part of the colon. The segment fails to pass on the peristaltic wave

Clinical manifestations:
1 Vomiting
2 Constipation – failure to pass meconium or infrequent loose stools
3 Abdominal distension, with bilious vomiting
4 Visible peristalsis

Diagnosis:
1 Abdominal X-ray shows dilated colon with narrowed distal segment
2 Rectal biopsy

Complications: Intestinal obstruction

Management: Temporary colostomy followed by resection of aganglionic segment at 9–12 months of age

Prognosis: Good with surgery

Imperforate or ectopic anus

Many types of abnormalities. In females the commonest type is displacement forward so that the anus opens in the vulva or vagina. Rectovaginal fistulas often occur. In the male rectovesical and rectourethral fistulas are found
Management: Surgery

Exomphalos (omphalocoele)

A herniation of abdominal contents through the umbilical ring. May rupture during delivery. Other complications include bowel infection, peritonitis, and intestinal obstruction. Managed surgically

Umbilical hernia

Very common in normal children and an operation to replace the viscera and repair the hernia may be necessary

Prune belly syndrome

Very rare, absence of abdominal muscles usually in male produces wrinkled appearance of the abdominal wall
Complications: Urinary tract infection, hydronephrosis, renal failure and pneumonia

CLINICAL FEATURES OF GASTROINTESTINAL DISEASE

Vomiting

Persistent vomiting may result from either medical or surgical problems.

Medical problems include:
1 Sucking and swallowing difficulties
2 Gastroenteritis
3 Sepsis
4 Meningitis
5 Urinary tract infection
6 Necrotizing enterocolitis
7 Drug withdrawal
8 Kernicterus
9 Adrenogenital syndrome
10 Inborn errors of metabolism such as galactosaemia and fructose intolerance

Surgical problems include:

1 Oesophageal atresia (presents early)

2 Intestinal atresia

3 Volvulus

4 Hirschsprung's disease

5 Pyloric stenosis (usually presents after the neonatal period)

6 Hiatus hernia

7 Malrotations and long duplications

Diarrhoea

Causes:

1 Without blood:
   a Gastrointestinal infection
   b Systemic infection
   c Disacharridase deficiency
   d Cow's milk protein intolerance
   e Drug-induced, e.g. antibiotics, ferrous sulphate, calcium gluconate

2 With blood:
   a Gastrointestinal infection: *Shigella, E. coli*
   b Necrotizing enterocolitis

Complications:

1 Dehydration:
   a Dryness of tongue and mucous membranes
   b Sunken anterior fontanelle
   c Reduced tissue turgor
   d Oliguria

2 Shock

3 Hypokalaemia

4 Hypernatraemia and hyperosmolarity

5 Predisposition to infection

Causes of abdominal distension

1 Gastrointestinal causes:
    a Intestinal obstruction
    b Sepsis
    c Necrotizing enterocolitis
    d Paralytic ileus
    e Perforation of a viscus
    f Swallowed air

2 Organomegaly:
    a Hepatomegaly: Haematoma; rubella syndrome, biliary atresia
    b Kidney enlargement: Hydronephrosis, polycystic kidneys, Wilms' tumour
    c Adrenals: Neuroblastoma
    d Splenomegaly: Rubella syndrome, haemolytic anaemia, infection

3 Ascites:
    a Hydrops fetalis
    b Peritonitis
    c Cardiac failure

Differential diagnosis of an abdominal mass

1 Unilateral mass:
    a Hydronephrosis
    b Tumours
    c Renal vein thrombosis
    d Horseshoe kidney
    e Adrenal haemorrhage or tumour
    f Ovarian cyst
    g Liver or gall bladder masses

2 Bilateral masses:
    a Polycystic kidney disease
    b Renal vein thrombosis

Investigation of an abdominal mass:

1 Full blood count, urea and electrolytes, urine analysis

2 Abdominal ultrasonography

3 Erect and supine abdominal X-ray

4 Renal scan

5 Intravenous pyelogram

6 Venous and arterial angiography

Causes of excessive weight loss

1 Inadequate intake:
   a Underfeeding
   b Difficulty in feeding

2 Vomiting:
   a Intestinal obstruction
   b Functional disturbance

3 Diarrhoea

4 Excessive surface evaporation

5 Diuresis:
   a Temporary congenital diabetes
   b Diabetes insipidus
   c Loss of oedema

NECROTIZING ENTEROCOLITIS

Pathophysiology: A disorder of uncertain aetiology which may result from ischaemia and infection of the bowel (usually the terminal ileum and colon) as a result of a hypoxic stress in a low birth weight infant. Occurs in about 1% of premature infants

Risk factors: The most important risk factors are previous umbilical artery or vein catheterization and exchange transfusion; others include:

1 Presence of hypoxic stress
   a Neonatal asphyxia
   b Respiratory distress syndrome
   c Sepsis

2 Compromised gut blood flow
   a Patent ductus arteriosus
   b Hypovolaemia; shock
   c Anaemia; exchange transfusion

3 Infection

4 Types of feeding: Hyperosmolar bottle feeds. Necrotizing enterocolitis is rare in breast-fed babies

Clinical features:
1 Progressive lethargy

2 Temperature instability

3 Bloody diarrhoea

4 Bleeding tendency

5 Pallor and shock

6 Peritonitis

7 Vomiting; may be bile-stained

8 Abdominal distension or ileus; absent bowel sounds

9 On abdominal X-ray:
   a Pneumoperitoneum
   b Intramural gas
   c Gas in the portal vein
   d Ring shadows

10 With severe disease, apnoea, hypotension, hypothermia and jaundice may result

Investigations:
1 X-rays (including upright or lateral decubitus)

2 Cultures (stool, blood, urine, CSF)

3 Arterial pH, P_{CO_2}, P_{O_2}

4 Serum electrolytes, calcium, bilirubin

5 Urine specific gravity

6 Stool Haematest

7 Haematocrit, white blood count

8 Platelet count

9 Clotting studies

Treatment:
1 General
   a Frequent physical examination (2–4 h), X-rays
   b Nothing orally for at least 10 days; intravenous feeding
   c Nasogastric suction

2 Infection: Antibiotics

3 Circulation
   a Blood pressure: correct hypotension
   b Urine output, specific gravity
   c If evidence of poor perfusion transfuse blood

4 Respiratory monitoring
   a Maintain PO_2
   b Maintain haematocrit
   c Acid–base monitoring

5 Coagulation status – platelets, etc.

6 Treatment of patent ductus arteriosus, if any

7 Hyperalimentation

8 Indications for surgery
   a Perforation
   b Deterioration of clinical course
   c Peritonitis

Prognosis:
1 25–50% mortality in those infants where perforation occurs

2 10% mortality in those infants who do not perforate
3 10% of infants will develop a recurrent episode of necrotizing enterocolitis

14

Neonatal and Perinatal Mortality

Definitions

1 Stillbirth: Babies delivered after the 28th week of gestation that fail to breath and/or show any sign of life. It is expressed per 1000 total (live and still) births. Stillbirths must be notified in the same way as live births to the Area Medical Officer

2 Perinatal mortality rate: The infant death rate calculated from the sum of stillbirths and 1st week neonatal deaths, per 1000 registered total births

3 Neonatal death rate: The infant death rate under 4 weeks after birth

4 Infant mortality rate: The number of deaths of all children under a year per 1000 live births

Causes of perinatal mortality

Between 1958 and 1970 the British perinatal mortality rate fell from 33:1000 to 23:1000. Social and geographical factors are involved. In Sweden the perinatal mortality rate is 12.1:1000. Some of the major causes are shown below (with percentages of total deaths in parentheses):
1 Prematurity (15–25%)

2 Congenital malformations (19%)

3 Hypoxia at any stage in or after the pregnancy, including respiratory distress syndrome (34%)

4 Birth injury (12–16%)

5 Rhesus haemolytic disease (3–5%)

6 Infection (1–4%)

7 Others

Factors that influence perinatal mortality

1 Geographic: e.g. higher mortality in the north and west of the UK

2 Age of mother: Higher mortality if the mother is over 30 years

3 Parity: First, and babies beyond the third, at greater risk

4 Social class: Mortality increases with descending social class

5 Past obstetric history: In particular, history of:
   a Previous abortions
   b Perinatal deaths
   c Premature labour

6 Antenatal care and place of delivery (an efficient health service)

7 Gestational age and birth weight
   a 'Safest' period of delivery is between 37th and 41st weeks
   b More than 50% of perinatal deaths are in babies with birth weights below 2.5 kg, especially if they are 'small-for-dates' babies

8 Pre-eclampsia and eclampsia

9 Breech presentation and delivery

10 Antepartum haemorrhage

11 Excessively long or short labours

12 Teratogenic drugs

Factors that have decreased the perinatal mortality rate

1 Improved standards of antenatal care

2 Better standards of living

3 Special care of low birth weight babies (in SCBUs)

4 Antenatal detection of high-risk groups, e.g. spina bifida

5 Prevention of Rhesus haemolytic disease

6 Active resuscitation of asphyxiated and hypoxic infants

THE SUDDEN INFANT DEATH SYNDROME

The sudden infant death syndrome (SIDS), or cot death, is the sudden death of any infant or young child which is unexpected according to the history and in whom a post-mortem examination fails to demonstrate an adequate cause of death. It causes about a third of all deaths in infants between 1 week and 1 year. It is the most common cause of death in this age-group.

Despite recent advances in developmental physiology, the cause of death remains unknown.

Highest rates are found in some areas in the UK and the lowest in Sweden:

Location	Rate per 1000 live births
Stockholm	0.06
Netherlands	0.42
Sheffield	2.1
Northern Ireland	2.5
Glasgow	2.7
Oxford Region	2.78
Grimsby and Cleethorpes	4.37

Epidemiological factors in SIDS:
1   Infant:
    a   Age 2–14 months
    b   Male more frequently affected
    c   Low birth weight
    d   Multiple births
    e   Family history
    f   Minor illness in week before death
    g   Bottle-fed
    h   Poor health and care
    i   Failure of clinical follow-up

2   Mother:
    a   Age <20 years
    b   High parity
    c   Poor antenatal care
    d   Obstetric complications
    e   Father's age <25 years
    f   Smoking
    g   Drug dependency

3   Environment:
    a   Winter
    b   Midnight to 9 a.m.
    c   Social class IV and V
    d   Non-whites
    e   Associated with regional occurrence of respiratory disease

Possible aetiology:
1   Respiratory:
    a   Anatomical abnormalities
    b   Infanticide
    c   Laryngospasm
    d   Nasal obstruction
    e   Suffocation
    f   Chronic hypoxia
    g   Abnormal reflexes

h Sleep apnoea
i Abnormal surfactant

2 Metabolic:
  a Cortisol insufficiency
  b Disorder of calcium metabolism
  c Subclinical amino acid disorder
  d Chronic metabolic acidosis

3 Cardiac:
  a Conduction disturbances
  b Lethal arrhythmias
  c Electrolyte imbalance

4 Immunological:
  a Anaphylaxis
  b Inadequate immune mechanisms
  c Overwhelming infection

5 Nutritional

6 General:
  a Overheating
  b Hypothalamic dysfunction
  c Nitrous fumes from domestic gas cooking and fires
  d Hypothermia
  e Hypoglycaemia

Prevention:

1 Improvements in antenatal care
2 Encouragement of breast-feeding
3 Raising the standard of care for infants
4 Improved health education

15

Diagnostic and Therapeutic Procedures

Cardiovascular

1 Blood drawing:
  a Capillary blood:
    i Warm the extremity and cleanse the skin with alcohol
    ii Use lateral side of heel and avoid previous sites
    iii Puncture with a stilette
  b Catheter blood samples from umbilical artery or radial artery
  c Venous blood: This is obtained from veins at the back of hand or scalp and from antecubital veins or external jugular veins

2 Intravenous infusion:
  a Scalp vein infusion:
    i Shave and cleanse the skin around the area chosen
    ii Place a light rubber band tourniquet around the head proximal to the vein, or place finger proximal to site to distend vein
    iii Flush needle with saline, and, leaving the syringe attached, insert needle tangentially into the vein

    iv Secure butterfly with plaster of Paris

  b Foot and ankle veins:

    i Cleanse the skin

    ii Restrain infant

    iii Cannulate the saphenous vein on the medial side of the ankle

3 Arterial puncture: This is necessary for the evaluation of acid–base and respiratory status of the infant, and requires collection of a blood sample which has not been exposed to air in any way. The syringe should be just slightly heparinized and during the procedure the inspired PO_2 should be held constant. Either the radial or temporal artery may be used, but when employing the radial artery the ulnar collateral artery should be tested by occluding the radial artery and making sure that the palm does not become pale

  a Radial artery:

    i Use high-intensity light source to visualize the radial artery, or locate by palpation

    ii Enter the artery at an angle of 20–30° and withdraw needle until the syringe starts to fill

  b Temporal artery:

    i Shave head

    ii Use small needle

    iii Straighten artery by finger tension

    iv Enter artery, withdraw needle slowly until syringe starts to fill

  c Brachial artery may also be used

Sources of error when performing arterial punctures include:

  a Failure to draw blood: Either the artery had not been entered, or it has been compressed accidentally

  b Venous sample: Venous pressure will not move

plunger. However do not assume dark blood is
venous

c   Air bubbles in sample will cause erroneous
reading

After needle puncture apply 10 min of firm pressure
to the artery

Complications:

a   Local ischaemia
b   Traumatic aneurysm
c   Haemorrhage

4   Exchange transfusion: During procedure check blood
pressure, heart rate and temperature and blood
sugar

a   Sterile precautions and gowns as for an
operative procedure. Infant should have had nil
by mouth for 4 h prior to the procedure; otherwise the stomach should be empty

b   Restrain infant under heat source

c   Assemble two three-way taps in series to connect
syringe, donor blood, waste container for
infant's blood and umbilical catheter

d   Catheterize the umbilical vein. Connect stopcock
to catheter and draw blood for measurement of
pretransfusion levels of bilirubin, haemoglobin,
serum protein, electrolytes etc. Monitor central
venous pressure (CVP) and electrocardiogram
(ECG)

e   Now remove and replace blood at a maximum
rate of around 4 ml kg^{-1} min^{-1}. Give 1 ml of
calcium gluconate per 100 ml of blood exchanged

f   Save final sample for post-exchange blood
measurements. Measure CVP. Monitor infant
closely for 2–4 h post-exchange.

Indications include:

a   Rhesus and other blood group incompatibility
b   Hyperbilirubinaemia

    c Sepsis

Complications of exchange transfusion:

    a Infections
    b Haemorrhage
    c Necrotizing enterocolitis
    d Perforations of vessels, peritoneum, or bowel
    e Hypervolaemia
    f Electrolyte abnormalities
    g Cardiac arrhythmias
    h Thrombocytopenia
    i Air embolus
    j Acidosis or alkalosis
    k Citrate intoxication
    l Hypoglycaemia
    m Hypothermia
    n Massive haemolysis caused by old exchange blood
    o Transient ileus

5 Vascular catheterization:

Types:

    a Umbilical artery catheters – easy and stable route

       i Indications:
- Respiratory distress syndrome (RDS) especially in low birth weight infants
- An immature infant with a birth weight of less than 1 kg
- Any severely ill infant requiring intensive care

      ii Procedure:
- Sterile technique – umbilical cord and surrounding area are carefully prepared with an antiseptic solution and infant's abdomen is draped with sterile towels
- The cord should be cut cleanly with a

scalpel and the two arteries identified
- The closed tip of iris forceps or an artery dilator is inserted into the lumen of an artery and a polyvinylchloride catheter filled with heparinized saline is threaded into the artery
- The catheter is introduced into the abdominal aorta and fixed in place (confirmed by X-ray examination) with a purse-string suture around the umbilicus. Tip of the catheter is usually at, or just above, the level of the diaphragm
- Keep catheter adequately flushed with heparinized fluid

iii Complications:
- Thrombotic problems
- Abdominal distension
- Blood in stools; necrotizing entero-colitis
- Decreased femoral pulses
- Haematuria

b Umbilical vein catheterization: This is indicated for intravenous fluid infusion or for exchange transfusions if there are no other peripheral veins available
Procedure:
- The infant is securely restrained, and the umbilical stump cleansed with anti-septic
- Cut the cord using a scalpel about 1 cm above the skin. This should disclose two thick-walled umbilical arteries and one large vein
- Holding the vein with forceps on either wall, the catheter previously filled with heparinized saline can be gently

introduced and secured, for attachment to an intravenous infusion set
  c Radial artery catheters

Urological

1 Clean – catch urine specimen
  a In male infants: Wash penis and foreskin and apply urine collection bag
  b As soon as infant urinates, transfer contents of bag into sterile container
  c Not a preferred method for female infants

2 Urethral catheterization:
  a In female infants: Cleanse external genitalia, while inserting catheter
  b Not the preferred method in male infants

3 Suprapubic bladder puncture:
  a Carefully cleanse skin with iodine and alcohol
  b Check that bladder is full
  c Palpate pubic bone
  d Place needle in midline superior to pubic tubercle
  e Carefully slide in needle attempting to withdraw piston aiming at infant's coccyx
  f If no urine obtained when needle is 3 cm inserted, then the bladder is empty

4 Cystography:
  a Catheterize and fill bladder with radiopaque medium under sterile conditions
  b Take anteroposterior, right and left oblique radiographs
  c Remove catheter – take films during and after voiding
  d Indicated in suspected bladder pathology or suspected vesico-ureteric reflux.

5 Intravenous pyelography:
  a Indications include:
    i One proven urinary tract infection
    ii Pyuria
    iii Haematuria
    iv Abdominal mass
    v Poor growth
    vi Pyrexia of unknown mechanism
    vii Congenital malformations
  b Obtain flat abdominal film. Insert radiopaque material intravenously
  c Precaution: Hypersensitivity may occur to contrast media – antihistamines and other anti-anaphylactic drugs may be required

6 Renal ultrasound

7 Renal scan

8 Renal biopsy: Indicated only in specialized circumstances

Neurological

1 Lumbar puncture: This is the safest method for obtaining cerebrospinal fluid (CSF). Indications include meningitis, suspected subarachnoid haemorrhage, unexplained seizures or apnoea.
  a Precautions: Exclude signs of raised intracranial pressure: check optic fundi
  b Apparatus: Short bevelled needle (20–21 gauge) with stylet; manometer with three-way tap, sterile drapes and gloves
  c Place infant either on his or her side or in a sitting position with the lower spine curved
  d Prepare a sterile field and drape with towels. A No. 21 needle with a stylet is inserted in the midline in the space between the 3rd and 4th lumbar spinous processes

> e Advance the needle *slowly* in the direction of the umbilicus and withdraw the stylet frequently to detect presence of CSF
> f Collect fluid into three tubes – about 0.5 ml in each tube
> g Examine fluid for turbidity and colour and send tubes to laboratory for cell count, Gram-staining, culture and sensitivity, glucose and protein estimations

2 Subdural puncture: This technique is rarely indicated
> a Shave and cleanse anterior two-thirds of scalp in the region of the anterior fontanelle
> b Drape with towels
> c Introduce 20–23 gauge (with stylet) needle in the mid-pupillary line through the coronal suture
> d Advance the needle slowly and remove the stylet frequently
> e When the dura yields, the needle is in the subdural space, and if fluid is present it should run out
> f Collect fluid into several tubes for cell count culture, glucose and protein determination, and for microbiological investigation

3 Cisternal puncture: This is a potentially risky procedure and is only indicated in extreme circumstances, and lumbar puncture is preferable wherever possible.

Respiratory

1 Intubation: Immediately after delivery of the head the infant's pharynx is aspirated with a large-bore soft PVC catheter. If the infant does not breathe by 30 s after birth ventilation is accomplished in most cases by bag and mask. If there are no respiratory movements after 1 min or the heart rate is below 100

beats/min the infant is intubated. Intubation for assisted respiration is also indicated under circumstances of respiratory distress (see Chapter 7)
Procedure:

a   Infant is placed supine and the neck should be partially extended

b   The laryngoscope is held in the left hand and passed into the right side of the mouth and then to the midline sweeping the tongue out of the way

c   The tip of the blade is advanced over the epiglottis and then withdrawn slightly so as to pass the epiglottis against the roof of the tongue and reveal the glottis

d   The endotracheal tube held in the right hand is inserted between the vocal cords to about 2 cm below the glottis

e   Check the position of the tube by auscultation of the chest. Fix the tube in place with adhesive tape

f   Apply intermittent positive pressure ventilation (IPPV) at a pressure of 30 cmH$_2$O and a rate of 40 times/min with an anaesthetic bag or using a Resuscitaire

g   A fine catheter is used to aspirate secretions in the tube

h   The stomach should be emptied using a feeding tube

i   IPPV should be stopped every 3 min for about 10–15 s to establish presence or absence of spontaneous respiration

j   Extubation. Apply suction to the airway both through and around the tube. Loosen all the tape so the tube may be pulled out smoothly as the infant reaches a full inspiration

Complications:

a   Injury to teeth, lips, tongue, epiglottis, arytenoid cartilages, aryepiglottis folds, vocal cords

    b Subcutaneous emphysema
    c Mediastinal emphysema
    d Pneumothorax
    e Infection
    f Reflex laryngospasm

2 Continuous positive airways pressure (CPAP): CPAP is used in the spontaneously ventilating patient in order to apply a continuous distending force to the alveoli.

Indications:
    a Infants with severe respiratory distress syndrome
    b Recurrent apnoea
    c Pulmonary oedema
    d Weaning off ventilator

Contraindications:
    a Pneumothorax
    b Pneumomediastinum
    c Congenital lobar emphysema

Procedure: The infant may be attached to CPAP by nasal prongs, face mask, head hood or by endotracheal tube:
    a Begin with about 6 cmH$_2$O to the airway depending on infant size, and if the infant still shows further respiratory distress, increase the pressure by 2 cmH$_2$O increments. However pressure should not be raised above 10 cmH$_2$O
    b Begin with an inspired O$_2$ content of 60%
    c Once patient improves, lower inspired O$_2$ content slowly, and reduce the airway pressure

Complications:
    a Keep high gas flow rate to prevent CO$_2$ rebreathing
    b Pneumothorax
    c Apnoea
    d Interference with venous return

3 Mechanical ventilation:
Indications:
  a Severe apnoea
  b Cardiorespiratory failure
Procedure:
  a Infant may be attached via endotracheal tube, nasotracheal tube, face mask, or body enclosure. Endotracheal tube is most common method of attachment
  b Settings of ventilator have to be adjusted according to patient's age, size and condition
  c Patient should be continuously monitored for blood gases, ECG, temperature and blood pressure

4 Emergency tracheostomy:
  a *This should be avoided whenever possible.* Thus an ordinary (14 gauge) injection needle pushed through the cricothyroid membrane should allow sufficient time for endotracheal intubation, and may be tried first
  b Indications for tracheostomy include:
    i Prolonged tracheal airway required, e.g. in congenital anomalies of the larynx or upper trachea, CNS disorders, etc.
    ii Foreign bodies – when removal is not possible via the larynx
    iii When endotracheal intubation is not possible due to either oedema or laryngospasm
Method:
  a With the neck of the infant slightly extended, make a horizontal incision below the cricoid cartilage and above the isthmus of the thyroid gland
  b Push the neck muscles laterally until the tracheal ring is exposed

    c Make a vertical incision through the 4th and 5th tracheal rings; through this introduce and secure the tracheostomy tube

    d Secure haemostasis, and obtain anteroposterior and lateral chest X-rays to check the position of the tracheostomy tube

Gastrointestinal

1 Tube feeding
Indications:
    a Small premature or very ill infants with inadequate sucking or swallowing reflexes
    b Congenital abnormalities that preclude sucking, e.g. choanal atresia, cleft palate
Procedure:
    a Introduce a feeding tube to a length of tube approximately equal to the distance between the nose of the infant and the xiphisternum
    b Draw back syringe to aspirate gastric contents – to ensure tube is in the stomach and not the trachea
    c Fill syringe attached to tube with feed and allow to enter stomach by gravity

16

Fluids and Electrolytes

Fluid and electrolyte therapy can be considered under the following subheadings:

1 Maintenance of daily requirements of fluid and electrolyte therapy

2 Correction of any imbalances caused by a particular illness

3 Replacement of continuing losses over and above those in (1)

4 Treatment of the underlying cause of the imbalance

MAINTENANCE

The daily requirements of fluid and electrolytes are determined by the level of losses per day.

The sources of water loss are:

1 Insensible water loss by evaporation from skin and respiratory tract

2 Water loss through the kidneys

3 Sweating – will vary with the environmental temperature.

4 Gastrointestinal – this may increase with, for example, diarrhoea

207

The degree of water lost is most reliably expressed as referred to unit surface area. In the neonate the ratio of surface area to weight is large, and so the water loss can be high relative to the size of the infant

Typical values of rates of water loss per day are:
  1 Insensible loss $500 \, ml/m^2$
  2 Minimal renal loss $500–800 \, ml/m^2$
  3 Sweat and gastrointestinal loss $200 \, ml/m^2$

Hence the maintenance water require-
ment is about $1.5 \, litre/m^2$

Note that the figures will vary. Thus:
  1 Insensible loss increases by 12% per degC of elevation of body temperature
  2 Renal loss – will vary with urine output
  3 Water loss through sweat – will increase with environmental temperature

Interconversion factors:

	mg/100 ml to mmol/l	mmol/l to mg/100 mg
Cl^-	× 0.285	× 3.5
K^+	× 0.257	× 3.9
Na^+	× 0.435	× 2.3

Bicarbonate: as cc bound carbon dioxide/100 ml (vol %) to HCO_3^- mmol/l: multiply by 0.447
HCO_3^- mmol/l to CO_2 cc/100 ml: multiply by 2.23

Protein: g/100 ml plasma to protein anion mmol/l: multiply by 2.43

Sodium chloride: 1 g contains 17 mmol Na^+ and 17 mmol Cl^-

Potassium chloride: 1 g contains 13 mmol K^+ and 13 mmol Cl^-

Sodium bicarbonate: 1 g contains 12 mmol Na^+ and 12 mmol HCO_3^-

A molar solution of a substance contains the molecular weight in grams of that substance in 1 litre.

Osmolarity denotes the molar concentrations per unit volume of all osmotically active particles in a solution.

Osmolarity of a substance which ionizes in solution = molarity × number of particles per mol resulting from ionization.

Taking into account the principal cations and uncharged organic constituents, the normal osmolarity of plasma is:

$$
\left.
\begin{array}{l}
Na^+\ (mmol/l) \quad\quad \times\ 2 \simeq 280 \\
+\ K^+\ (mmol/l) \quad\quad \times\ 2 \simeq\ \ 8 \\
+\ \dfrac{urea\ (mg/100\ ml)}{60} \times 10 \simeq\ \ 5 \\
+\ \dfrac{glucose\ (mg/100\ ml)}{180} \times 10 \simeq\ \ 5
\end{array}
\right\} \simeq 298\ mosmol
$$

Useful data

About: 75% of the infant's body weight is water

45% of the infant's body weight is intracellular water

30% of the infant's body weight is extracellular water

8% of the infant's body weight is whole blood

4% of the infant's body weight is plasma

Electrolyte requirements (per day):

1 Sodium: 2–4 mmol/kg

2 Potassium: 1–3 mmol/kg

3 Chloride: 2–4 mmol/kg

FLUID AND ELECTROLYTE IMBALANCES

Dehydration

1 Assessment of the degree of dehydration
  This is made clinically employing the following features:
  a Weight loss – this is useful if the dehydration is acute; any loss over 10% of body weight is regarded as moderate to severe dehydration
  b Clinical features:
    i Behaviour – infant is irritable in mild to severe dehydration but may become lethargic if dehydration is severe
    ii Skin turgor is diminished on dehydration; the skin may also be pale or grey
    iii Depressed fontanelles; sunken eyes
    iv Cardiovascular features – pulse may be elevated. Fall in blood pressure is a late sign
  c Investigations:
    i Blood indices: Changes in haematocrit and blood urea
    ii Urine: Changes in urine output and urine specific gravity
  Dehydration can be classified according to parallel changes occurring in plasma osmolarity into isotonic, hypotonic and hypertonic dehydration. Since the major extracellular fluid ion is Na^+, we can use the terms isonatraemic, hyponatraemic, or hypernatraemic respectively, as basically sodium is the ion responsible.

2 Isotonic dehydration:
  a Pathophysiology. Net electrolyte and water loss is isotonic:
    i Osmolarity of remaining extracellular fluid is unchanged
    ii There is no intracellular–extracellular water redistribution, and so

    iii Only the extracellular fluid compartment is altered

    iv Serum sodium is normal

b Causes. Fundamentally due to a fluid loss only involving the extracellular space, e.g.:

    i Peritonitis

    ii Volvulus

    iii Low intestinal obstruction

    iv Burns

    v Intussusception

c Management: Fundamentally, to restore the extracellular fluid volume, using a balanced salt solution

3 Hypotonic dehydration:

a Pathophysiology: The overall loss of water and electrolytes is hypertonic. Hence there will be a net fall in extracellular fluid osmolarity. This causes water to leave the extracellular fluid compartment to enter the intracellular fluid compartment, and this has the following consequences:

    i The fall in volume of the extracellular fluid is greater than the actual volume of water lost

    ii The additional decrease in extracellular fluid volume corresponds to an increase in the intracellular fluid volume

    iii The plasma sodium will *fall* below around 130 mmol/l

b Management: The basic principles of management are:

    i Correct the extracellular fluid deficit by using a balanced salt solution

    ii Correct the sodium deficit. This can be calculated from the normal value of the total body water, and the serum sodium, but often corrects itself through continuation of administration of a balanced salt solution, or of normal saline

4 Hypertonic dehydration
  a Pathophysiology:
    i The overall loss of water and electrolyte is hypotonic. This results in an increased osmolarity of the remaining extracellular fluid. Hence water will shift from the intracellular to the extracellular fluid, and this decreases the net extracellular fluid deficit
    ii Serum sodium is elevated (150 mmol/l or more)
    iii This form of dehydration can also occur with administration of excess electrolytes to a patient with isotonic or even hypotonic dehydration
  b Management: Since the extracellular fluid volume loss is moderated by its shift from the intracellular space, restoration of the extracellular fluid volume is often not an immediate priority. The correction should be performed with a *gradual* infusion of hypotonic electrolyte solution, since the electrolyte deficit is relatively small, monitored by following any rise in blood pressure very closely.

ACID–BASE PROBLEMS

In simple terms, plasma pH is a function of the ratio of the plasma HCO_3^- concentration to the CO_2 pressure. It may be altered as a result of either metabolic or respiratory disturbances.

  1 Pathophysiology: Arterial blood findings in the different types of alkalosis or acidosis are as follows:

	pH	HCO₃⁻	PCO₂
Metabolic acidosis	Decreased	Decreased	Decreased
Respiratory acidosis	Decreased	Increased	Increased
Metabolic alkalosis	Increased	Increased	Increased
Respiratory alkalosis	Increased	Decreased	Decreased

In general, if the net acid–base imbalance is predominantly metabolic in nature, changes in pH, HCO_3^- and arterial PCO_2 take the same direction and the main alteration is in the level of HCO_3^-. In contrast, if the disturbance is predominantly respiratory in origin, changes in HCO_3^- and arterial PCO_2 are opposite to the change in pH, and the main alteration is in the PCO_2

Adverse effects of acidosis include:

  a   Myocardial depression

  b   Increased pulmonary vascular resistance with right to left shunting

  c   Depressed cerebral and cellular metabolisms

2   Metabolic acidosis. This may result from:

  a   Loss of HCO_3^-, for example through the gastrointestinal tract

  b   Addition, or production, of strong acid – this tends to utilize bicarbonate ion as buffer – for example, in the accumulation of lactic acid secondary to hypoxic changes in intestinal volvulus

     Metabolic acidosis will be partly compensated for by the following physiological mechanisms:

    i   Buffer systems, which remove H^+ – for example, haemoglobin and phosphate

    ii   Respiratory compensation – hyperventilation will decrease the arterial PCO_2. This will decrease the change in the HCO_3^-/PCO_2 ratio

    iii   Renal mechanisms – the kidneys will

excrete acid (e.g. as NH_4^+) and so generate
HCO_3 to replace the HCO_3^- lost

Causes of metabolic acidosis include:
  a Hypoxia
  b Shock
  c Infection
  d Diarrhoea
  e Cardiac failure
  f Renal failure
  g Renal tubular acidosis
  h Aminoacidosis

3 Respiratory acidosis: This results from increased
arterial PCO_2 due to decreased alveolar ventilation.
Ultimately this results in a fall in blood pressure and
tissue hypoxia due to depressed cardiac output and a
fall in the peripheral resistance. Physiological com-
pensatory mechanisms include an increased
generation of HCO_3^- by buffering and by the kidneys,
which also excrete increased acid.
Causes include:
  a Asphyxia
  b Respiratory depression
  c Respiratory distress syndrome
  d Pneumonia

4 Metabolic alkalosis: This is the result of an effective
increase in HCO_3^-. It may result from:
  a Administration of an excessive amount of HCO_3^-
  b Loss of hydrogen ions from the extracellular
     fluid space
  c Hypokalaemia
Physiological compensation mechanisms are:
  a Extracellular fluid buffers – these can liberate
     H^+
  b Respiratory mechanisms – decreased alveolar
     ventilation will increase the arterial PCO_2. This

partly corrects the change in the HCO_3^-/PCO_2 ratio

c Renal mechanisms excreting HCO_3. These, however, will be affected by the following:

  i In the presence of a depletion of the extracellular space, there is increased Na^+ reabsorption in both the proximal and in the distal tubules. In the proximal tubule, HCO_3^- is reabsorbed with the Na^+, and in the distal tubule, H^+ is exchanged for Na^+

  ii In the presence of hypokalaemia (see below), the threshold for HCO_3 reabsorption increases. Hence H^+ shifts into the tubule cell and is secreted, resulting in an *acid* urine, even though the blood is alkaline

  iii In the presence of elevated arterial PCO_2, there is an increase in the renal threshold for HCO_3^-

5 Respiratory alkalosis: This results from a fall in arterial PCO_2, due to hyperventilation. Physiological mechanisms that compensate for it are:

a Buffering – these will liberate H^+, and thereby reduce the HCO_3^-

b Renal mechanisms – these result in a fall in the production of HCO_3^-, and in the net acid excretion of H^+

Note that respiratory alkalosis will result in a decrease in the level of ionized calcium, as this tends to bind to un-ionized plasma protein. This causes neuromuscular irritability, with exaggerated reflexes, and even tetany.

6 Management of acid–base imbalance

a Management of the underlying cause is a high priority

b Management of any volume or osmolarity disorder will facilitate the intrinsic regulatory mechanisms in restoring pH balance

c Direct management of the pH disorder is indicated if this is severe. In practice only acidosis need be managed, using a solution of sodium bicarbonate with dose calculated by nomogram. Where there is a concurrent danger of Na^+ overload, tris-hydroxyaminomethane (THAM) may be used instead as a neutralizing buffer.

Potential complications of sodium bicarbonate administration:

i Hyperosmolality

ii Intracranial haemorrhage

iii Hypernatraemia

iv Cellular dehydration

v Tissue necrosis

vi Increased P_{CO_2}

REPLACEMENT OF CONTINUING FLUID LOSS

This is considered under the following headings:

1 Determining the losses

2 Replacement fluids used

3 Replacing the losses

1 Determination of continuing fluid loss: Losses through the gastrointestinal tract. The volumes of the fluids should be measured daily, and their electrolyte content assessed. Typical compositions include:

a Gastric fluid:

H^+	40– 60 mmol/l
Na^+	30– 70 mmol/l
K^+	5– 15 mmol/l
Cl^-	100–150 mmol/l

b Bile:

Na^+	110–150 mmol/l

$$K^+ \qquad 5-\ 15\,mmol/l$$
$$Cl^- \qquad 80-120\,mmol/l$$
$$HCO_3^- \qquad 30-\ 50\,mmol/l$$

c Pancreatic juice:

$$Na^+ \qquad 110-140\,mmol/l$$
$$K^+ \qquad 5-\ 15\,mmol/l$$
$$Cl^- \qquad 50-\ 80\,mmol/l$$
$$HCO_3^- \qquad 80-120\,mmol/l$$

d Small bowel:

$$Na^+ \qquad 100-150\,mmol/l$$
$$K^+ \qquad 5-\ 15\,mmol/l$$
$$Cl^- \qquad 90-150\,mmol/l$$
$$HCO_3^- \qquad 20-\ 50\,mmol/l$$

e Diarrhoeal stools – very variable:

$$Na^+ \qquad 40-\ 70\,mmol/l$$
$$K^+ \qquad 20-\ 60\,mmol/l$$
$$Cl^- \qquad 20-\ 60\,mmol/l$$

2 Replacement fluids used: The overall composition of the fluids being given should be similar to that of the fluids lost, e.g. gastric juice may be replaced by infusion of a solution of around $90\,mmol/l\ Na^+$, $40\,mmol/l\ K^+$ and $130\,mmol/l\ Cl^-$.

3 Replacing the loss:

a Replacement therapy should be made in the light of daily blood electrolyte levels, with possibly also analysis of the electrolyte content of the fluid being lost. Particular care must be taken to avoid hyperkalaemia

b Losses should not be allowed to run ahead of replacement, which should cover each 6–8 h period (or even less)

SPECIFIC ELECTROLYTE PROBLEMS

These include:

1 Hypokalaemia; potassium depletion

2 Hyperkalaemia

3 Hyponatraemia
4 Hypernatraemia } (see also Dehydration, above)

5 Imbalances in divalent cation – calcium, magnesium (see Chapter 11)

1 Hypokalaemia:
Causes:
   a Inadequate K^+ intake
   b Alkalosis
   c Diarrhoea and vomiting
   d Iatrogenic – diuretics and steroids
Clinical features: May not be marked even in severe hypokalaemia. Depressed deep tendon reflexes, vague muscle weakness and hypotonia.
Investigation:
   a Serum K^+ below 3.0 mmol/l. Note that dehydration may mask an overall depletion of K^+
   b ECG: Signs below may not be unique to K^+ depletion:
      i Prolonged Q–T interval
      ii T wave inversion
      iii ST segment depression
      iv P wave inversion
      v Ventricular extrasystoles
Management: Correction should be gradual – over a few days, to avoid the danger of hyperkalaemia. Normally, not more than 3 mmol/kg of K^+ should be administered per day. The deficit should be estimated at the onset, and the daily requirement plus up to 5 mmol/kg per day should be administered. The potassium may be administered orally, with the water intake, or intravenously, using solutions that contain 20–40 mmol/l K^+

2 Hyperkalaemia:
Causes include:
   a Excessive K^+ intake

b Acidosis
c Shock and oliguria
d Haemolysis during blood sampling
e Adrenal insufficiency
f Chronic renal failure

Clinical features:
a Often asymptomatic
b If severe – listlessness, confusion, bradycardia, shock, cardiac arrest

Investigation:
a Serum potassium above 6 mmol/l
b Electrocardiogram:
   i peaked T wave
   ii prolonged QRS
   iii increased P–R interval
   iv irregularities of rhythm; heart block

Management: Severe hyperkalaemia is a medical emergency. It should be managed promptly, under monitoring of serum K^+ and ECG

a Withhold K^+ intake
b Give insulin and glucose
c Give 10% calcium gluconate intravenously
d Consider measures to eliminate K^+:
   i K^+ – free ion exchange resins either by enema or by mouth
   ii Peritoneal or haemodialysis

3 Hyponatraemia; sodium depletion
Causes include:
a Diarrhoea and vomiting
b Iatrogenic – intravenous fluids; diuretics; indomethacin therapy
c Intestinal obstruction
d Congestive cardiac failure
e Sepsis
f Renal failure

    g Inappropriate secretion of antidiuretic hormone
       due to asphyxia, brain damage and meningitis

4 Hypernatraemia
   Causes include:
    a Dehydration (see above)
    b Diarrhoea and vomiting
    c Intestinal obstruction
    d Osmotic diuresis; hyperglycaemia
    e Iatrogenic
    f Congenital adrenal hyperplasia

Bibliography

Avery, G. B. (1981). Neonatology: Pathophysiology and Management of the Newborn, 2nd Edn. (Philadelphia: Lippincott)

Avery, M. E. and Fletcher, B. D. (1974). The Lung and its Disorders in the Newborn Infant, 3rd Edn. (Philadelphia: W. B. Saunders)

Behrman, R. E. (1977). Neonatal–Perinatal Medicine: Diseases of the Fetus and Infant, 2nd Edn. (St Louis: C. V. Mosby)

Chiswick, M. L. (1978). Neonatal Medicine. (London: Update Books)

Cockburn, F. and Drillien, C. M. (1974). Neonatal Medicine. (Oxford: Blackwell Scientific Publications)

Davies, R. A., Robinson, R. J., Scopes, J. W., Tizard, J. P. M. and Wigglesworth, J. S. (1972). Medical Care of Newborn Babies. Clinics in Developmental Medicine, 44/45 (London: Spastics International Medical Publications and Heinemann Medical)

Dawes, G. S. (1968). Foetal and Neonatal Physiology, Year Book Medical Publishers.

Dubowitz, L. M., Dubowitz, V. and Goldberg, C. (1970). Clinical assessment of gestational age in the newborn infant, J. Pediatr., 77, 1

Egan, D. F., Illingworth, R. S. and McKeith, R. C. (1971). Developmental Screening 0–5 years. Clinics in Developmental Medicine, 30. (London: Spastics International Medical Publications and Heinemann Medical)

Forfar, J. O. and Arnell, G. C. (Eds.) (1978). Textbook of Paediatrics. (Edinburgh: Churchill Livingstone)

Goodwin, J. W. et al. (1976). Perinatal Medicine. (Baltimore: Williams and Wilkins)

Gunter, M. (1973). Infant Feeding. (Harmondsworth: Penguin Books)

Hey, E. (1971). The care of babies in incubators, Recent Advances in Paediatrics (Eds.) Gairdner, D. and Hull, D. (Edinburgh: Churchill Livingstone)

Hill, R. M. (1979). Perinatal Pharmacology. (Evansville, Indiana: Mead Johnson)

Hirata, T. and Brady, J. P. (1977). Newborn Intensive Care: Chemical Aspects. (Springfield, Ill.: Charles C. Thomas)

Illingworth, R. S. (1979). The Normal Child, 7th Edn. (Edinburgh: Churchill Livingstone)

Keay, A. J. and Morgan, D. M. (1978). Craig's Care of the Newly Born Infant, 6th Edn. (Edinburgh: Churchill Livingstone)

Kelnar, G. and Harvey, D. (1980). Intensive Care of the Newborn. (London: Macmillan)

Klaus, M. H. and Fanaroff, A. A. (1979). Care of the High-risk Neonate, 2nd Edn. (Philadelphia: W. B. Saunders)

Klaus, M. H. and Kennele, J. H. (1976). Maternal–Infant Bonding. (St. Louis: C. V. Mosby)

Korones, Sheldon B. (1981). High Risk Newborn Infants, 3rd Edn. (St. Louis: C. V. Mosby)

Lissauer, T. (1981). Neonatal resuscitation. Hosp. Update, 7, 109

Lorber, J. (1972). Spina Bifida Cystica (Myelomeningocoele). Results of treatment of 270 consecutive cases with criteria for selection for the future. Arch. Dis. Childh.

O'Doherty, Neil (1979). Atlas of the Newborn. (Lancaster: MTP Press Ltd)

Redo, S. Frank (1976). Principles of Surgery in the First Six Months of Life. (New York: Harper-Medical)

Redo, S. Frank (1978). Atlas of Surgery in the First Six Months of Life. (New York: Harper-Medical)

Rickham, P. P. and Irving, Irene M. (1978). Neonatal Surgery, 2nd Edn. (London: Butterworths)

Rowe, Richard D. et al. (1981). The Neonate with Congenital Heart Disease, 2nd Edn. (Philadelphia: W. B. Saunders)

Salmon, M. A. (1978). Developmental Defects and Syndromes. (Aylesbury: H. M. and M. Publications)

Schaffer, A. J. and Avery, M. E. (1977). Diseases of the Newborn, 4th Edn. (Philadelphia: W. B. Saunders)

Smith, C. A. and Nelson, N. M. (1976). The Physiology of the Newborn Infant, 4th Edn. (Springfield, Ill.: Charles C. Thomas)

Smith, D. W. (1976). Recognizable Patterns of Human Malformation, 2nd Edn. (Philadelphia: W. B. Saunders)

Strang, L. B. (1977). Neonatal Respiration. (Oxford: Blackwell Scientific Publications)

Valman, H. B. (Ed.) (1979). Paediatric Therapeutics. (Oxford: Blackwell Scientific Publications)

Vulliamy, D. G. (1977). The Newborn Child, 4th Edn. (Edinburgh: Churchill Livingstone)

Appendix

NORMAL NEONATAL VALUES

		Approx normal physiological range (SI units)
Sodium	136 –145	mmol/l
Potassium	4 – 5.5	mmol/l
Calcium	1.8– 2.9	mmol/l
Urea	2.5– 6.5	mmol/l
Haemoglobin	16 – 20	g/dl
Magnesium	0.6– 1.0	mmol/l
Bicarbonate	18 – 23	mmol/l
PaO_2	8 – 13	kPa
$PaCO_2$	4.3– 6.1	kPa
Glucose	2.0– 5.3	mmol/l
Protein	50 – 70	g/l
Platelets	150 –400	$\times 10^9$/l
WBC	9 – 30	$\times 10^9$/l
Thyroxine	5–14 days > 120	nmol/l
	14–28 days > 100	
Thyroid-stimulating hormone	<1–5.8	μU/l

MEAN WEIGHTS AT DIFFERENT AGES, FOR PRESCRIBING PURPOSES

Age	Weight (kg)	Range (kg)
Birth	3.2	2–4
1 month	4	3–5
2 months	4.5	4–6
4 months	6.5	5–7
6 months	8	6–10
9 months	9.5	7–11
12 months	10	8–12
18 months	11	9–14
2 years	12	10–15
3 years	15	12–18
4 years	16	14–20
5 years	18	15–22
6 years	20	16–24
7 years	23	17–30
8 years	25	18–34
9 years	28	31–37
10 years	30	23–40
11 years	36	25–46
12 years	39	26–50

DOSAGES OF COMMONLY USED DRUGS (DAY = 24 h)

Ampicillin
  Route: Oral, intramuscular, intravenous
  Dose: $100 \, mg \, kg^{-1} \, day^{-1}$

Cephaloridine
  Route: Intramuscular
  Dose: $35 \, mg \, kg^{-1} \, day^{-1}$

Chloramphenicol
  Route: Oral, intramuscular, intravenous
  Dose: $25–50 \, mg \, kg^{-1} \, day^{-1}$

Cloxacillin
  Route: Oral, intramuscular, intravenous
  Dose: 100 mg kg^{-1} day^{-1}

Colistin sulphomethate
  Route: Intramuscular
  Dose: 4–6 mg kg^{-1} day^{-1}
          (50 000–75 000 iu kg^{-1} day^{-1})

Erythromycin
  Route: Oral
  Dose: 25–40 mg kg^{-1} day^{-1}
  Route: Intravenous
  Dose: 10 mg kg^{-1} day^{-1}

Fusidic acid
  Route: Oral
  Dose: 20–40 mg kg^{-1} day^{-1}

Gentamicin (sulphate)
  Route: Oral
  Dose: 50 mg kg^{-1} day^{-1} (*not* absorbed)

Gentamicin (base)
  Route: Intramuscular
  Dose: 6 mg kg^{-1} day^{-1} (blood levels must be checked)
  Route: Intraventricular
  Dose: 1–2 mg per dose

Kanamycin
  Route: Intramuscular
  Dose: 15 mg kg^{-1} day^{-1}

Nystatin
  Route: Oral
  Dose: 100 000 units per dose (4 hourly)

Neomycin
    Route: Oral
    Dose: 50 mg kg^{-1} day^{-1}

Penicillin G
    Route: Intramuscular
    Dose: 240 000 units kg^{-1} day^{-1}

Penicillin V
    Route: Oral
    Dose: 60 mg kg^{-1} day^{-1}

Chloral hydrate
    Route: Oral
    Dose: 10–15 mg/kg per dose

Diazepam
    Route: Oral, intramuscular, intravenous
    Dose: 0.04–0.25 mg/kg once only

Paraldehyde
    Route: Intramuscular
    Dose: 0.1–0.2 ml/kg per dose

Phenobarbitone
    Route: Intramuscular
    Dose: 3 mg/kg per dose 12 hourly
    Route: Oral
    Dose: 5 mg kg^{-1} day^{-1}

Phenytoin
    Route: Intramuscular
    Dose: 3 mg/kg per dose 12 hourly

Route: Oral
Dose: 5 mg kg^{-1} day^{-1}
Route: Intravenous
Dose: 8 mg/kg slowly once

Calcium gluconate 10%
  Route: Intravenous
  Dose: 1.0 mg/kg per dose (100 mg/kg per dose)
          0.2 ml/kg per dose for tetany
          2–4 ml kg^{-1} day^{-1} for maintenance in hypo-glycaemia

Digoxin
  Route: Oral, intramuscular
  Digitalizing dose (safe dosage for newborn):
    0.02 mg/kg once
    0.01 mg/kg 8 hourly twice
  Maintenance:
    less than 1 week old: 0.01 mg/kg daily
    more than 1 week old: 0.02 mg/kg daily
    reduce dose by 30% in pre-term infants

Ferrous sulphate
  Route: Oral
  Dose: Below 2.5 kg: 30 mg twice daily
         Above 2.5 kg: 60 mg twice daily

Frusemide
  Route: Oral
  Dose: 2 mg/kg once daily
  Route: Intramuscular, intravenous
  Dose: 1 mg/kg once daily
         Potassium supplements may be needed

Naloxone
  Route: Intramuscular, intravenous
  Dose: 0.02 mg/kg per dose

EFFECTS OF DRUGS ON THE FETUS

Drugs should not be given to pregnant women unless absolutely
necessary

Drug	Possible effects on the fetus
Androgens and progestagens	Virilization in female fetus; neoplasm in vagina (not manifest until adolescence)
Antineoplastic drugs	Deformities
Antithyroid drugs	Goitre; hypothyroidism
Chloroquine	Deafness; corneal opacities
Corticosteroids	Adrenal atrophy
Cortisone	Cleft palate
Ethanol (in large amounts)	Fetal alcohol syndrome; growth-retardation
Folic acid antagonists	Deformities
Rifampicin	Neural tube defect
Streptomycin	Deafness
Sulphonylureas	Hypoglycaemia
Tetracycline	Discolouration of teeth
Thalidomide	Phocomelia
Warfarin	Nasal bone hypoplasia

DRUGS THAT MAY AFFECT BREAST MILK COMPOSITION

Drugs where harmful effects have been reported:

Amantadine	Iodine
Antineoplastics	Kanomycin
Anthraquinone	Lithium
Atropine	Phenindione
Bromides	Potassium iodide
Carbimazole	Primidone
Cascara	Streptomycin
Chloramphenicol	Sulphonamides
Cortisone	Tetracycline
Diazepam	Thiouracil
Ergotamine	

Drugs where doubt remains as to safety:

Barbiturates	Phenylbutazone
Erythromycin	Prednisolone
Isoniazid	Prednisone
Meprobamate	Propranolol
Methyldopa	Reserpine
Metronidazole	Thiazide diuretics
Nalidixic acid	Warfarin

ADVERSE EFFECT OF DRUGS

System	Drug	Adverse effects
Cardiovascular	Digoxin	Bradycardia
	Prednisolone	Hypertension
Haematological	Cytotoxic agents } Chloramphenicol	Bone marrow depression
	Co-trimoxazole } Phenytoin	Megaloblastic anaemia
Metabolic	Frusemide	Hypokalaemia
	Prednisolone	Hyperglycaemia
	Thiazides	
Neurological or neuromuscular	Phenobarbitone } Antihistamines	Drowsiness
	Phenytoin } Carbamazepine	Ataxia
	Metoclopramide	Dystonia
	Prochlorperazine	Hyperkinesis
Gastrointestinal	Most drugs	Nausea and/or vomiting
	Ampicillin	Diarrhoea
	Ampicillin	Monilial infection
	Aspirin	Gastric bleeding
	Tetracyclines	Stained teeth
Cutaneous	Ampicillin } Phenytoin	Rash
	Penicillin	Urticaria
	Prednisolone and glucocorticoids	Cushingoid syndrome

WEIGHT CENTILES FOR GESTATIONAL AGE

A weight below the 10th centile is deemed light-for-dates and above the 90th large-for-dates.

Completed week from LMP	Centiles of birth weight (kg)		
	10th	50th	90th
32	1.40	1.99	2.65
33	1.68	2.28	2.93
34	1.94	2.53	3.18
35	2.17	2.76	3.40
36	2.37	2.96	3.60
37	2.54	3.13	3.77
38	2.68	3.27	3.90
39	2.79	3.38	4.01
40	2.87	3.46	4.10
41	2.93	3.51	4.15
42	2.95	3.54	4.18

For firstborn infants 150 g should be added to the weight before using the table. The difference in weight between girls and boys is not of practical significance. (From Thomson, A. M., Billewicz, W. Z. and Hytten, F. E. (1968). *J. Obstet. Gynaecol. Br. Commonw.*)

HEAD CIRCUMFERENCE CENTILES FOR GESTATIONAL AGE

Completed week from LMP	Centiles of head circumference (cm)		
	10th	50th	90th
32	28.4	30.0	31.2
33	29.2	30.8	32.2
34	30.0	31.6	33.0
35	30.8	32.4	33.6
36	31.4	33.0	34.2
37	32.0	33.4	35.0
38	32.6	34.0	35.6
39	33.2	34.6	36.2
40	33.6	35.0	36.8
41	34.2	35.6	37.2
42	34.6	36.2	37.8

(From Babson, S. G. (1970) *J. Pediat.*)

CONVERSION NOMOGRAMS

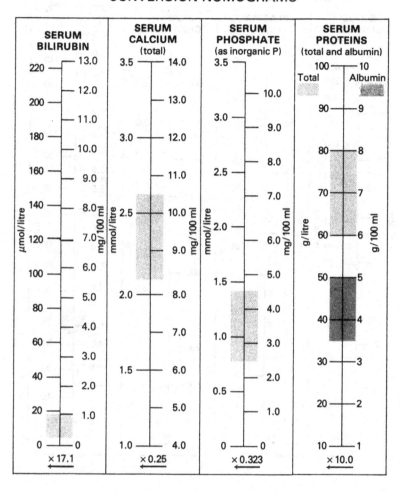

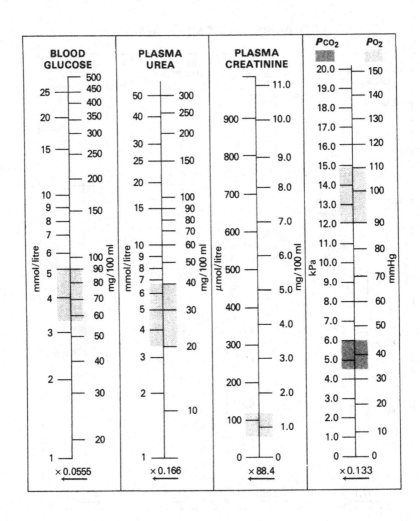

Index

233